B Main CT Scans
Be n Clinical Practice

Brain CT Scans in Clinical Practice

Usiakimi Igbaseimokumo

With 109 Figures, 50 in Full Colour

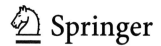
Springer

Usiakimi Igbaseimokumo
Division of Neurosurgery
University of Missouri School of Medicine
University Hospitals & Clinics
Columbia MO
USA
igbas@aol.com

ISBN 978-1-84882-364-8   e-ISBN 978-1-84882-365-5
DOI 10.1007/b98343
Springer Dordrecht Heidelberg London New York

British Library Cataloguing in Publication Data
A catalogue record for this book is available from the British Library

Library of Congress Control Number: 2009920533

Printed on acid-free paper

Springer is part of Springer Science+Business Media
(www.springer.com)

Preface

Across emergency rooms all over the world, thousands of patients are referred for brain CT scans daily. A radiologist often has to interpret the scan or a consultation has to be made to a neurosurgeon to review the scan. Most of this happens late at night and is a significant source of discontent. Thus having frontline physicians to be proficient in interpreting the emergency brain CT scan improves the efficiency of the whole pathway of care and is potentially life saving as time is of the essence for many patients with severe brain injury or stroke.

Underlying all of the above and the primary reason for writing this book is because the skill required to determine *an immediate life threatening abnormality* in a brain CT scan is so basic and can be learned in a short time by people of various backgrounds and certainly by all physicians. 'Indeed the emergency head CT scan is comparable to an electrocardiogram in usefulness and most definitely as easy to learn.' This book is therefore written for caregivers the world over to demystify the emergency CT brain scan and to empower them to serve their patients better. It is obvious to me from the response from people I have had opportunity to teach this subject that not only is there a desire to learn this basic skill but also people learn it quickly and wonder why it has not been presented so simply before.

It is to fulfil this need and to reach a wider number that I have put together these basic, proven steps in the interpretation of emergency brain CT scan for ER physicians, primary care physicians, medical students and other primary care givers.

Foreword

Interpretation of the emergency CT brain scan is a visual art. Comparison is made between the image in front of you and a reference image. For the experienced person, this reference image is imprinted in the mind, therefore comparison is quick. For the beginner, you can either carry several examples of every possible appearance of normal and abnormal scans to compare with or read this book! This book contains a few proven ways of quickly learning to interpret a brain CT scan, irrespective of your previous experience.

The radiologist's experience is related to the number of hours he or she has spent looking at CT scans. The radiologist conveys his evaluation of the CT scan in words that often come in a particular sequence and combination. This book is about helping you to rapidly understand and confidently use the same language used by the radiologist.

The difference is that whereas the radiologist aims for perfection, you aim for functionality. For instance it will be acceptable and clinically safe if an intern physician looks at the brain CT scan in Fig. 1 and can make a judgement of the urgent action required like ABCs (airway, breathing and circulation with c-spine) and *call a neurosurgeon immediately*. This is life saving and efficient without the need for a long list of differential diagnoses before deciding on this action. The skill to act decisively about the CT scan in front of you can be acquired in a very short time. And the author has reduced that time to less than one day using this book!

Korgun Koral, MD
Associate Professor of Radiology
University of Texas Southwestern

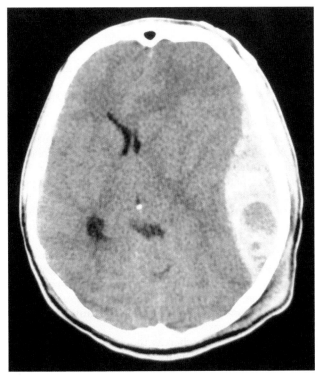

FIGURE 1. Emergency action required! ABCs and call Neurosurgeon!

Acknowledgements

My heartiest gratitude goes to my wife Ebitimi and my kids Gesiye, Ilayefa and Binaere who volunteered the real cost in time to prepare this book. My eternal gratitude to The Isouns – Professor Turner T. Isoun, PhD and Dr. Miriam J. Isoun, PhD – for spiritual, financial and intellectual support on this and every other project I ever embarked upon, thank you.

I would like to thank those who read the manuscript and made useful suggestions including especially my classmate and friend Dr. Eme Igbokwe, MD. I would also like to thank Dr. Korgun Koral, MD for finding the time to read the manuscript and making pertinent suggestions. Dr. Jim Brown, MD and Dr. Kristen Fickenscher, MD were a very present source of encouragement and critique.

I would like to acknowledge Stacy Turpins for the original drawings and the framing of the illustrations.

My sincere gratitude to Medical Modeling for the prototype of the cover image.

Lastly despite their best thoughts and efforts, any error remains singularly mine and please contact me with any suggestions.

Contents

Chapter 1
Introduction to the Basics of Brain CT Scan

THREE BASIC DENSITIES OR DIFFERENT SHADES OF GREY

The first secret is that we describe CT scan findings as '*densities*', of which there are three common easily identifiable ones to learn. 'In general the higher the density the whiter the appearance on the CT scan and the lower the density the darker the appearance on the brain CT scan.' The reference density (the one you compare with) is the brain, *usually* the largest component inside the skull. Anything of the *same* density as the brain is called ISODENSE, and it is characterised by a dull greyish white appearance (Fig. 1.1). *Thus the brain is the reference density*. Anything of *higher* density (whiter) than the brain is called HYPERDENSE, and the skull is the best example of a hyperdense structure that is seen in a normal brain CT scan. The skull is easily identified as the thick complete white ring surrounding the brain. Similarly, anything of *lower* density (darker tone) than brain is described as HYPODENSE.

The cerebrospinal fluid (CSF) is the typical example of a hypodense structure in the brain CT scan (Fig. 1.1). Air is also hypodense and surrounds the regular outline of the skull in CT, just as the air surrounds the head in life. Between the pitch formless *blackness* of air and the *greyish white* appearance of the brain, the cerebrospinal fluid presents a faint granular hypodense appearance, which may vary slightly but is identified by its usual *locations*. You will come to realise later that 'appreciating the usual locations of CSF is the key to understanding brain pathology on CT scan' (Igbaseimokumo 2005). We will come back to this idea later, but for now suffice it to say that the skull is highly whitish in appearance (Fig. 1.1) and is clearly identified as an oval white ring surrounding the brain. The brain is greyish white, and

U. Igbaseimokumo, *Brain CT Scans in Clinical Practice*,
DOI 10.1007/b98343_1, © Springer-Verlag London Limited 2009

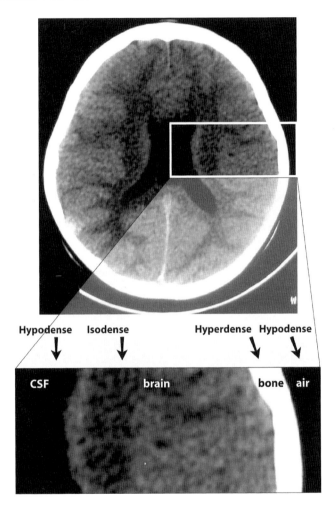

FIGURE 1.1. The different densities of CT scan.

the CSF is dark and faintly granular on close inspection (but not as dark as air) and has specific normal locations.

How to Identify an Abnormality on the CT Scan
Similar to the normal densities, abnormalities on the CT scan are also described simply as *high density, low density or the same density as brain.* So what could a hyperdense (high density) appearance on a CT scan represent? This is perhaps the one most

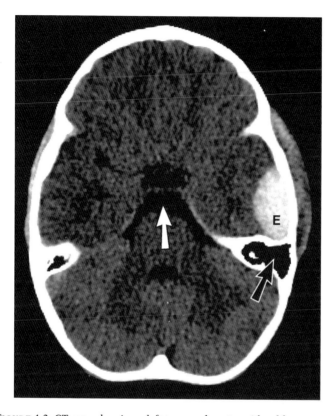

FIGURE 1.2. CT scan showing a left temporal acute epidural haematoma (E). Notice that the egg-shaped blood clot (E) has a density higher than brain but lesser than bone. Can you make out the boundary between the bone and the blood clot? Just behind the haematoma, the air in the mastoid (black arrow) is darker than the CSF in the centre of the brain (white arrow). The CSF has a faint granular hue on close inspection, which is absent in air.

important fact you will get to learn about CT scans. The answer is simple – ***blood*** is the most common hyperdense abnormality found on a brain CT scan (Fig. 1.2). So if a hyperdense appearance is not in the right location for bone then it must be *blood until proven otherwise*. So the rule of thumb is that 'anything white in the CT scan is either blood or bone'.

There are two common exceptions to the above rule. You might as well learn them now. The pineal gland is a little calcified

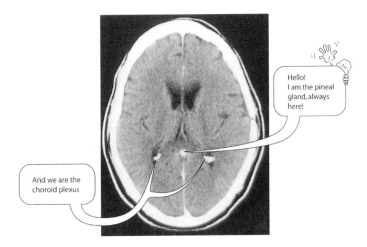

FIGURE 1.3. Brain CT scan showing pineal and choroids plexus calcifications.

speck in the middle of the CT scans of most adults. It is unmistakable after you see it a few times. Look at it smiling at you in Fig. 1.3.

The second exception is the calcified choroid plexus, which is located in the body of each lateral ventricle, lying indolently in the CSF like the Titanic at the bottom of the sea. Again they are so easily identified that you only need to see them once to remember (Fig. 1.3). So you can well assume at this stage that every other hyperdense lesion is abnormal. 'The important fact to take away is that most abnormalities will be hyperdense especially in the emergency setting.' Blood is the most common hyperdense lesion, and I will later on describe what a calcified tumour (the second-most common hyperdense lesion) looks like. However, the common hypodense lesions seen on a brain CT scan are directly related to increased *fluid* in the brain as in oedema from ischemic stroke (Chapter 3), tumours and infection (Chapter 5) and hydrocephalus (Chapter 4). We will come back to these later.

The Density of Blood Changes with Time!
Yes, the density of blood changes with time. You generally have bleeding inside the head from an injury such as a motor vehicle collision or a fall or burst blood vessels from high blood pressure. The blood is brightest on the first day of injury or bleeding and

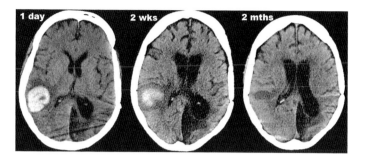

FIGURE 1.4. Note the change in the density of the blood from hyperdense (1 day) to hypodense with time (2 months).

from then on the density gradually fades. So in thinking about what you are seeing on the scan, it is important to remember how long after the injury or the onset of symptoms before the scan was done. This is an important idea that we will come back to later in the book but an example of what happens to the blood with time is shown in Fig. 1.4. In describing changes over time, the word ACUTE simply means recent onset whereas CHRONIC means something that has lasted for a long time.

SYMMETRY–MIRROR IMAGE

The next important fact will become apparent a lot quicker if you looked in a mirror (now!). Ok! If you do not have a mirror nearby, then try and recall the last time you looked in the mirror. For most of us: you had one ear, one eye, one nostril and *half a mouth* on either side of the face. In short the left and right sides of your face look nearly identical! Similarly, the brain CT scan consists of two identical halves (mirror images). There is a dividing line, which passes through the middle. Therefore if I give you one half of a CT scan (Fig. 1.5), you can actually recreate the other half, the mirror image!

So the great news is this: ***even if you have never seen a CT scan before, you can simply compare one half of the scan against the other half. If there are significant differences (for instance if the right and left halves are not the same), then the scan is abnormal*** (Fig. 1.6). If the right and left are identical on every slice then the image is said to be symmetrical and most *probably* normal (except in hydrocephalus where you can have symmetrical abnormality).

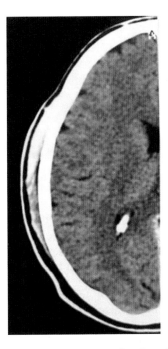

FIGURE 1.5. Half of the CT head (Can you sketch in the mirror image to show the choroids plexus and the ventricles and the skull?).

The following exercise will help drive home this very fundamental principle in learning to interpret brain CT scans. It includes normal and abnormal scans. *Note that by convention, the right side of the brain CT scan is on the left of the reader and it should be labelled as such (see chapter 2).*

Exercise 1: Can you pair-up the correct halves and mark which ones are abnormal?
Clue: One half of some of the pairs are enlarged. Focus on the pattern!

If you found the above exercise difficult **DO NOT WORRY!** Here is a simplified version showing an example of a normal scan with identical halves (mirror images) and one with significant abnormality on the opposite side. I hope you can say which side is abnormal!

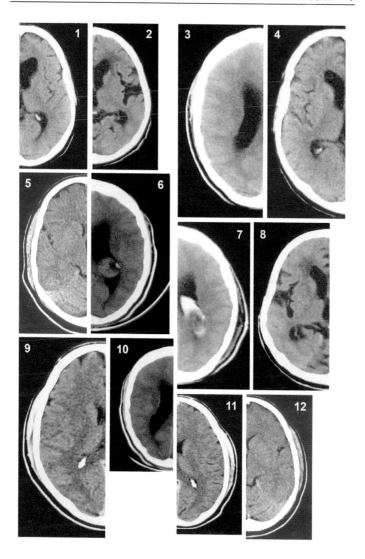

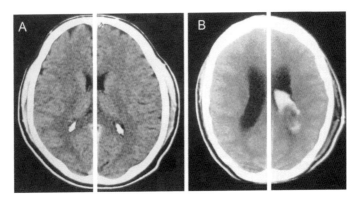

FIGURE 1.6. Brain CT scan with identical halves (A = normal scan) and an abnormal brain CT scan (B) showing blood clot in one half.

CEREBROSPINAL FLUID (CSF) SPACES – THE COMPASS OF BRAIN CT SCAN

The next important concept in understanding the brain CT scan is to identify the normal pattern of CSF spaces in the brain. The CSF spaces (low density) in Fig. 1.7A are large and easily identified. Examining the next two scans will show that the pattern is quite similar but the spaces are smaller, yet all these films will pass as normal for different ages.

Just as the faces of mankind differ in appearance, so do the CSF patterns of our brains. In general, the brain on the left belongs to a very elderly person with lots of CSF spaces due to shrinkage of the brain (atrophy), and the one on the right belongs

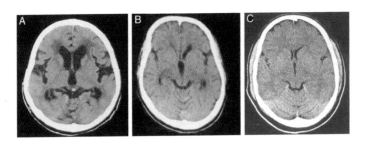

FIGURE 1.7. The pattern of CSF spaces in the brain.

to a young adult. However, the similarity in the shape of the CSF spaces is apparent on close inspection. This teaches us where to look if the fluid spaces are not immediately obvious: for instance, you look where you ought to find 'CSF' and see *if* it has been replaced by blood as in subarachnoid haemorrhage or squeezed out by tumour. In the next section, we will identify and name the different CSF spaces and also name the bony landmarks in the floor of the skull that relate to the CSF spaces.

IDENTIFYING ABNORMALITIES IN THE CSF SPACES

The CSF spaces are the clue to identifying abnormalities on the brain CT scan. They could be filled with blood and appear hyperdense (Figs. 1.8 and 1.9) or the CSF could be squeezed out by swelling of the brain (Fig. 1.10) or by tumour (Fig. 1.15). In either case knowing the usual location of the CSF spaces will help you to

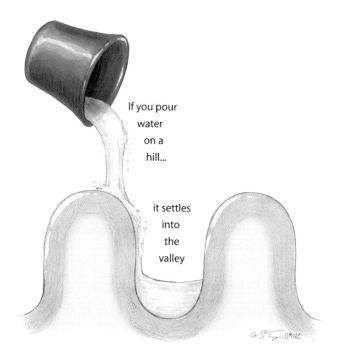

If you pour
water
on a
hill...

it settles
into
the
valley

FIGURE 1.8. (continued)

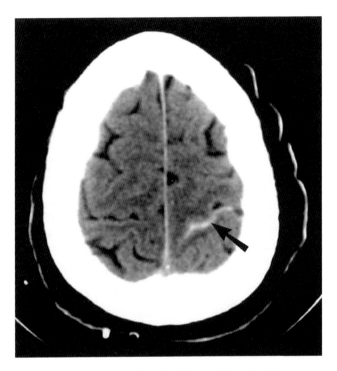

FIGURE 1.9. Brain CT scan of a 48-old-year old male following motor vehicle collision. It shows the hyperdense clot taking the place of CSF in the sulcus (black arrow). You can also see normal sulci that appear dark. The straight white line in the middle is the falx cerebri and the blood in the sulcus is the white density inclined lazily at 45 degrees to the falx cerebri (black arrow).

detect what is going on. We will examine a few large and *readily* identifiable ones and extend the same principles to less obvious cases.

FIGURE 1.8. (continued) If you pour water or blood on a hill it will settle in the valley. In the brain, the gyri are the hills and the sulci (which normally contain CSF) are the valleys, so the blood will settle in the sulci displacing the CSF; therefore instead of being dark, the sulci turn white. This is a fundamental principle you need to understand in looking for subarachnoid haemorrhage in CT scan, as in the real example below (Fig. 1.9).

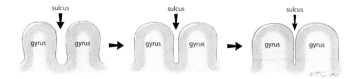

FIGURE 1.10. Schematic drawing showing how the sulci disappear as the gyri enlarge. In a real brain CT scan, the appearance changes from the image in Figs. 1.11 to 1.12.

BRAIN SWELLING

The next important concept is this: whenever the brain swells, it means the gyri get larger and the sulci get smaller as illustrated below:

As in Fig. 1.12, the sulci and gyri may not be obvious because of either swelling or compactness as in most young people. However, it is very important to appreciate that the whole brain surface is made of sulci and gyri, which is easier to appreciate in Figs. 1.11 and 1.13. 'All the gyri and sulci of the brain are named. Some of the CSF spaces are larger (big sulci) and more constant (present in every scan) and easily identified; therefore they are

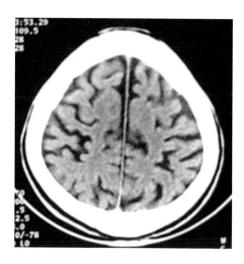

FIGURE 1.11. CT scan showing widely spaced CSF spaces. This and the next figure also serve to illustrate the point that although some CT scan images appear simply as a granular mass as in Fig. 1.12, you should bear in mind that it always represents sulci and gyri on the surface of the brain as in this figure.

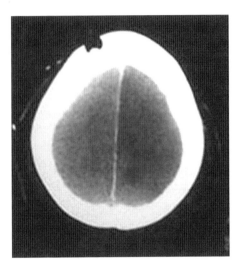

FIGURE 1.12. CT scan showing very tight, almost absent spaces due to swelling. This and Fig. 1.11 also serve to illustrate the point that although some CT scan images appear simply as a granular mass as in this figure, you should bear in mind that it always represents sulci and gyri on the surface of the brain as in Fig. 1.11.

used as the compass for navigating the maze of sulci on the surface of the brain (Fig. 1.13). Can you name some of them?'

Occasionally the presence of air (dark spots in Fig. 1.14A) in the sulci allows us to appreciate easily that the homogenous-looking appearance of the CT scan (Fig. 1.14) actually consists of sulci and gyri.

Brain Tumours
The sulci may also be obliterated by expanding lesions within the brain such as a tumour or an abscess. In addition to mechanical compression of the sulci, associated swelling of the surrounding gyri from oedema leads to the appearance of complete obliteration of the sulci as shown in Figs. 1.15 and 1.16.

EXTRA AXIAL AND INTRA AXIAL LESIONS

The type of lesion in Figs. 1.15 and 1.16 is called intra axial, meaning it is inside the brain itself. However, a mass lesion that arises in the coverings of the brain like a meningioma (tumour

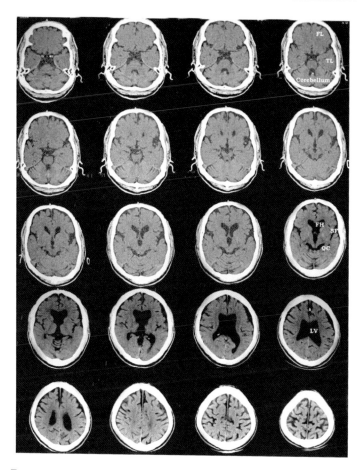

FIGURE 1.13. In the brain CT scan above, the CSF pattern is more obvious and I have named a few landmark structures for your ready reference (FL = frontal lobe; TL = temporal lobe; FH = frontal horn of lateral ventricle; SF = Sylvian fissure; QC = Quadrigeminal cistern; LV = lateral ventricle).

of meninges, Figs. 1.17 and 1.18), which will immediately squash both gyri and sulci together is called an extra axial mass. The schematic drawing (Fig. 1.17) is a general illustration of what happens to the brain with an extra axial mass. Similarly a blood clot on the surface of the brain or over the membranes of the brain will also be an extra axial lesion. Can you identify the

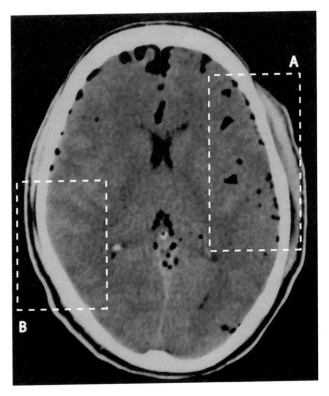

FIGURE 1.14. This 38-year-old male fell from a height at a construction site. He was comatose on admission with bilateral raccoon eyes. The brain in box B appears amorphous and granular while the brain in box A has the air (dark spots) outlining the sulci (A). 'It is important to emphasise that the air helps us to appreciate that the granular appearance in box B actually consists of gyri and sulci. *So interpreting a CT scan does call for imagination of how the CT image relates to the 3-dimensional human brain.*'

abnormality in the CT scan in Fig. 1.17? *'And do not forget the right half of the CT scan is on the left hand side of the reader!'*

BASIC ANATOMY OF THE BRAIN SURFACE

To summarise, we have learnt that the brain surface consists of gyri and sulci and that the sulci are normally filled with CSF,

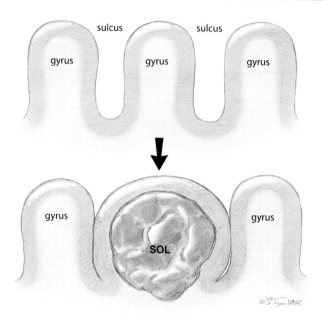

FIGURE 1.15. The term SOL stands for 'space occupying lesion'. This could be a tumour or abscess or blood clot, which occurs in the centre of the gyrus and expands outwards to squeeze the sulci.

which gets replaced by blood or is squeezed out by swelling of the brain from oedema or expanding masses (Figs. 1.15, 1.16, 1.17 and 1.18). Do not worry if you do not know where the CSF goes when it is squeezed, we will get there by and by. For now let us try and name the CSF spaces and some parts of the brain. Sounds ominous like a top-level course in neuroanatomy! Do not despair; I know it is not many people's favourite subject so we will keep it very simple. So let us start by naming some of the CSF spaces in Fig. 1.13. Let us look at the first row of four images, the left two of which are reproduced in Fig. 1.19.

The illustration in Fig. 1.20 shows that the brain is made up of gyri and sulci (gyrus and sulcus in singular form). The sylvian fissure you see in the picture above corresponds to the sylvian fissure we identified on the CT scan in Fig. 1.19. 'This fissure separates the frontal and temporal lobes, and it is the area through which the carotid arteries enter and supply the brain, and hence the place to look for blood when we are looking for

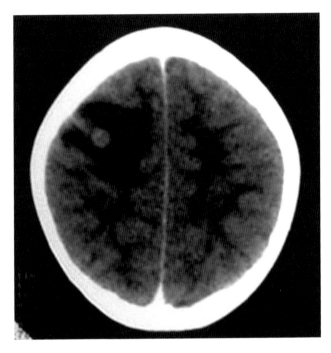

FIGURE 1.16. The right-sided small lesion and oedema are squeezing neighbouring sulci and gyri similar to the schematic illustration in Fig. 1.15. 'Note the low density of the oedema surrounding the lesion. The white matter normally appears less dense than the cortex as seen on the left hemisphere in this scan. It is referred to as grey white differentiation on the CT scan, but the oedema from the lesion is darker than the normal white matter low density and *it is not CSF.*'

evidence of subarachnoid haemorrhage (SAH).' This point will be clear when we get to the chapter on SAH, but you can see the obvious connection and the reason why this CSF space is important. *The sulci are roofed over by the arachnoid membrane (Chapter 2) to form the subarachnoid space, which is continuous throughout the brain surface hence blood can flow through these spaces to anywhere intracranially!* In Figs. 1.21 and 1.22, the sylvian fissure, the interhemispheric fissure and the subarachnoid spaces over the surface of the brain are filled with blood leading to failure of circulation of CSF, hence the hydrocephalus (enlarged

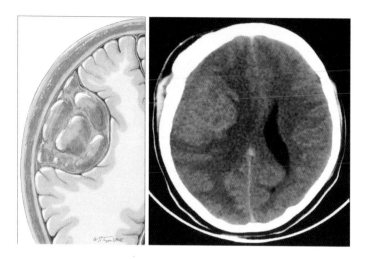

FIGURE 1.17. Drawing of the effects of an extra axial mass on the brain and a CT scan showing an ISODENSE mass. Using the principles we learnt earlier, can you detect asymmetry in the two halves of the scan? Can you make out where the tumour is? (Note = it is isodense with brain). Start first by working out which side has the abnormality and then look for the abnormality. Yes, you read correctly. First decide which side is abnormal, then look for the abnormality. *'(And this is the clue: whenever there is a pressure effect or mass effect, the CSF is the first thing to be displaced. If you think back in this chapter, we started with what distorts the sulci and progressed to what will distort the sulci and gyri. So in a CT scan, a general rule of thumb is that the half with the least amount of CSF is likely to be abnormal. That goes without saying if the CSF is the most easily displaced component of the cranium, the lesion is likely to start displacing CSF from its immediate vicinity! So the left with the large dark CSF space is the normal side and the right without any CSF space is abnormal. Now can you make out the abnormality? It is isodense; for instance, same density as the brain so you will need your skills at pattern analysis to identify the abnormality. Use pencil and paper and sketch your impression of the tumour before you look at Fig. 1.18, which contains the contrast CT scan highlighting the tumour. We will come back to contrast enhancement in the chapter on tumours.)'*

ventricles – Chapter 4). Note that the pineal gland is just behind the top of the third ventricle as in Fig. 1.22.

These observations will conclude the introduction. Please revise the interactive portions of this chapter including the exercises.

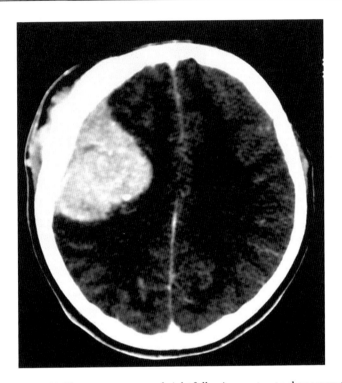

FIGURE 1.18. The tumour appears bright following contrast enhancement and you can gain the impression that the brain is squashed in all directions. I will like you to make one important observation on the opposite side to the tumour. You can see the uniform low density of the CSF in the ventricle and then the white matter and then the cortex with bright streaks in it before you reach the skull. 'You should make a mental note of the difference in density between the white matter next to the ventricle and the grey matter next to the skull. This is called grey white differentiation, a phrase that surfaces frequently, usually when this distinction is lost in severe brain oedema.'

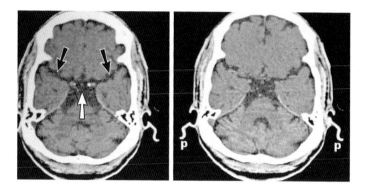

FIGURE 1.19. Right and left sylvian fissures (black arrows) meeting at the ***suprasellar cistern***. You can trace these narrow CSF pathways in each successive slice until they break up into small channels. 'It is present in every brain CT scan but not always visible due to variations in their sizes but you must look here for evidence of CSF distortion or subarachnoid haemorrhage! Outside the skull you can see the cartilage of the pinna (p), another important point of reference as you navigate the CT images.'

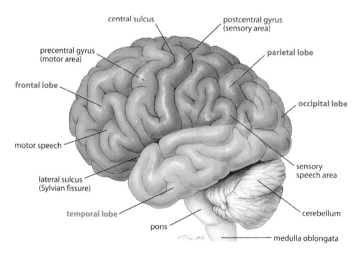

FIGURE 1.20. Pictorial illustration of the brain. Here is a reminder for those who have not recently graduated from a neuroanatomy course!

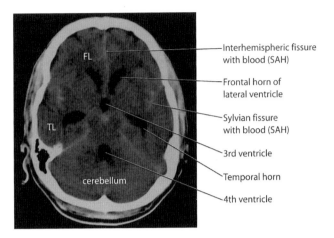

Interhemispheric fissure with blood (SAH)

Frontal horn of lateral ventricle

Sylvian fissure with blood (SAH)

3rd ventricle

Temporal horn

4th ventricle

FIGURE 1.21. CT scan showing subarachnoid haemorrhage (SAH) and hydrocephalus. Note how the sylvian fissure marks the boundary between the frontal lobe (FL) and the temporal lobe (TL) (compare with Fig. 1.20). The mirror image nature of brain CT scans (symmetry) is apparent in this illustration. The temporal horns are normally collapsed and not easily seen, so their enlargement in a CT scan is abnormal and the third ventricle is rounded instead of being slit-like. (See Chapters 3 and 4 for SAH and hydrocephalus, respectively).

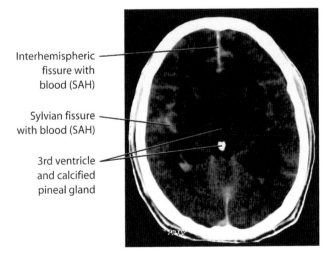

Interhemispheric fissure with blood (SAH)

Sylvian fissure with blood (SAH)

3rd ventricle and calcified pineal gland

FIGURE 1.22. CT scan showing subarachnoid haemorrhage in the CSF spaces. Note the difference in density between the calcified pineal gland (normal) and the blood in the Sylvian fissure and the interhemispheric fissure. Also note that the pineal gland is directly behind the third ventricle.

Exercise 2: Can you identify the CSF spaces the arrows are pointing to in this normal CT scan?

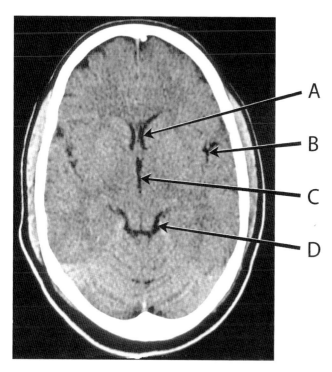

Answers to:

Excercise 1.
1 & 4; 2 & 8; 3 & 7; 5 & 12; 6 & 10; 9 & 11

Excercise 2.
A = Left frontal horn
B = Left sylvian fissure
C = Third ventricle
D = Ambient cistern

Chapter 2
Head Injury

INTRODUCTION – INTRACRANIAL HAEMATOMAS

From the last chapter we learnt that acute blood is hyperdense (whiter) compared to the brain. In this chapter we will use that information to identify the various lesions that can occur in the brain following trauma. Although diffuse injury is more common (Figs. 1.10, 1.12 and 1.14), the vast majority of emergency neuro-surgical intervention in trauma involves the evacuation of mass lesions like epidural and subdural haematomas as well as intracerebral haematomas; hence we will focus on identifying these lesions promptly. In Fig. 2.1, you should now be able to confidently identify the blood clots. The first thing to recognize is that the blood clot in each case is closely related to the skull. As a matter of fact, it is separating the brain from the skull. You will easily appreciate from further examination of the images that in Fig. 2.1A the clot is biconvex (acute epidural haematoma, EDH) whereas in Fig. 2.1B the clot is crescent shaped like a new moon draped over the surface of the brain (acute subdural haematoma, ASDH).

'In the majority of cases, this simple difference in shape accurately distinguishes an epidural haematoma from a subdural haematoma.' We will come back to this in more detail below. Your understanding of the conceptual (anatomic) basis for the difference in the CT appearance of these two lesions is not only important for your accurate use of the terms but '"epidural haematoma patients" behave significantly differently from patients with acute subdural haematoma, hence the distinction is important'.

U. Igbaseimokumo, *Brain CT Scans in Clinical Practice,*
DOI 10.1007/b98343_2, © Springer-Verlag London Limited 2009

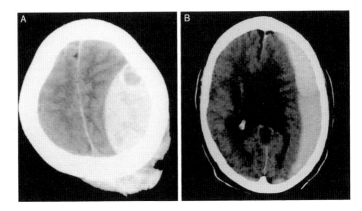

FIGURE 2.1. Non-contrast CT scan showing an acute epidural haematoma (with overlying scalp swelling) (A) and acute subdural haematoma (B).

Depressed skull fractures are easy to identify clinically and on the CT scan (Fig. 2.2), often signifying direct blow to the affected part of the skull. They could be associated with different kinds of brain haemorrhage as shown here. Linear fractures are less easy to see on the CT scan, and the 'bone window' (see Fig. 2.21A and B) is essential for their diagnosis.

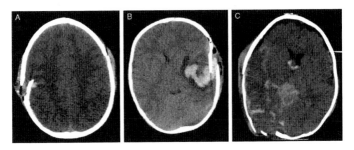

FIGURE 2.2. CT scan showing A: depressed skull fracture; B: depressed fracture and associated traumatic intracerebral haematoma and; C: Depressed fracture and associated traumatic SAH and contusions.

Acute, Subacute and Chronic Subdural Haematomas
The word 'acute' simply means recent, for instance that the blood is still white or hyperdense on the CT scan, as opposed to 'chronic' when the blood changes colour (density) to isodense or

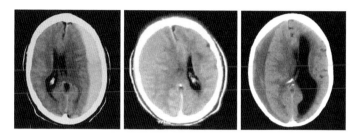

FIGURE 2.3. Showing acute (hyperdense), isodense chronic and hypodense chronic subdural haematomas, which represent three different stages of evolution (not the same patient). Clue – the side with less CSF is abnormal.

hypodense at about three weeks from the trauma. It represents the natural evolution of all haematomas.

THE BRAIN COVERINGS (MENINGES) AND THE SUBARACHNOID SPACE

The word '*sub*dural' simply means *below* or *under* the dura, and *extra*dural or *epi*dural simply means *outside or above* the dura. Figure 2.4 illustrates the layers of the brain and Fig. 2.5 graphically illustrates the naming (classification) of blood clots as epidural or subdural. In simple terms, the classification is based on whether the clot is above or below the dura.

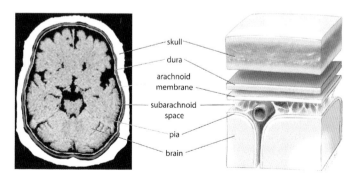

skull
dura
arachnoid membrane
subarachnoid space
pia
brain

FIGURE 2.4. Schematic illustration showing the different layers covering the brain.

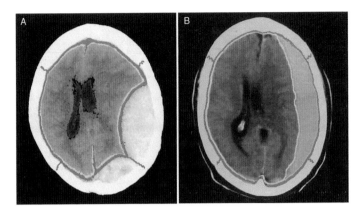

FIGURE 2.5. Schematic illustration showing the difference between acute epidural haematoma (A) and acute subdural haematoma (B). Can you confidently distinguish the AEDH from the ASDH? Notice that the thick dura mater inserts into the skull and delimits the potential free expansion of the epidural haematoma.

Note particularly that the dura is a tough relatively thick membrane, and it is illustrated as the red layer under the *skull*. If the blood collects between the skull and the dura then it is called an epidural haematoma as it is outside the dura. The next layer is the arachnoid membrane illustrated by the light blue colour which in life is transparent and flimsy (very much like cling film), and it lines the inner surface of the dura; thus a *potential* space exists between the arachnoid and the dura. This is called the subdural space, which is normally collapsed in life but when bleeding occurs into this space it is called a subdural haematoma (see Figs. 2.3 and 2.5).

Further examination of Fig. 2.4 shows that the third layer to cover the brain is the pia mater, which in fact tightly hugs the brain going into every valley (sulcus) and mound (gyrus) that makes up the surface of the brain. It is illustrated by the pink layer in Fig. 2.4. Since the arachnoid does not hug the brain tightly but bridges over the sulci, a relatively large space is formed between the arachnoid and the pia. This space is *filled with CSF* and since it is below the arachnoid, it is called the subarachnoid space (Fig. 2.4). Bleeding into this space is called subarachnoid haemorrhage (Figs. 1.8, 1.9, 1.21 and 1.22) (see also Chapter 3).

The last layer covering the brain is the pia mater. Blood clots or tumours in the brain deep to the pia mater are called intraaxial and those outside the pia mater are called extra axial. This distinction is important when we talk about tumours and even haematomas. The image in Fig. 2.6 illustrates a traumatic intracerebral haematoma, for instance inside the brain (within the pia mater). Again notice that the ventricle on that side is squashed and that is called mass effect, for instance pressure from the clot squeezing the surrounding brain and displacing the CSF.

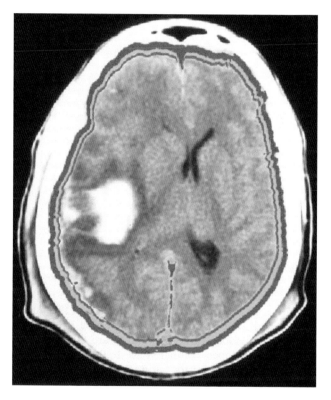

FIGURE 2.6. CT scan showing traumatic intracerebral haematoma – within the parenchyma of the brain – for instance inside the pia mater.

THE PARTS OF THE SKULL AND NAMING OF HAEMATOMAS

The skull is the ultimate covering of the brain and because epidural haematomas in particular are often named after the skull bone, that they are lying under it is important to remind ourselves of the parts of the skull. The bones of the skull are illustrated in

Fig. 2.7, and they are joined at their margins by saw-teeth joints called sutures, where the dura inserts very firmly into the skull (Figs. 2.5 and 2.7).

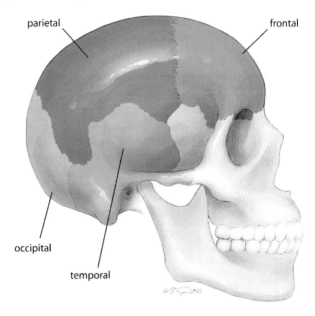

FIGURE 2.7. Parts of the human skull.

This diversion into anatomy is important because the lobes of the brain roughly correspond to the portion of the skull they relate to as well. For instance, the frontal lobe of the brain is under the frontal bone of the skull and so are the parietal, temporal and occipital lobes (compare Figs. 1.20 and 2.7). The dural insertions into the skull (at the sutures) leave very deep impressions on the skull, which are readily evident as in this picture of the interior of the skull (Fig. 2.8). The coronal suture separates the frontal bone from the parietal bone and the lambdoid suture separates the parietal bone from the occipital bone.

'Epidural haematomas do not normally cross these suture lines as the dura insertion is tough thereby restricting the enlarging clot to the confines of the sutures of that particular bone, hence they enlarge like a balloon and compress the brain and appear biconvex.'

It is important therefore to appreciate that epidural haematomas are biconvex in appearance because the dura is fixed (inserted firmly into the skull Fig. 2.9) at the sutures whereas

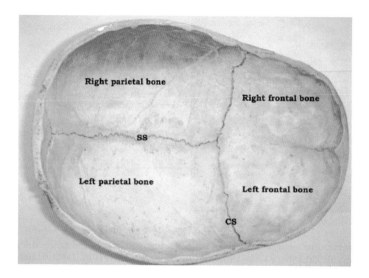

FIGURE 2.8. Interior view of the skull showing some of the dural insertions (sutures). (CS = coronal suture; SS = sagittal suture).

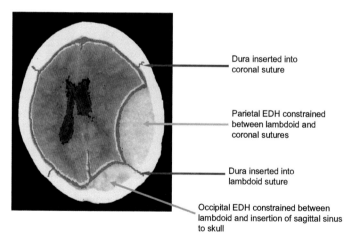

FIGURE 2.9. CT scan with line drawings showing the dural insertions and epidural haematomas restricted by the sutures.

the subdural space is continuous over the surface of the brain, hence acute subdural haematomas (Fig. 2.10) and chronic subdural haematomas (Fig. 2.11) spread over the surface of the brain and assume a crescent shape.

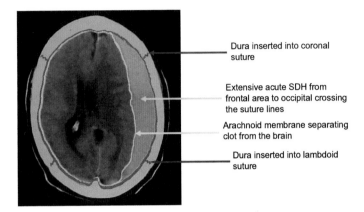

Dura inserted into coronal
suture

Extensive acute SDH from
frontal area to occipital crossing
the suture lines

Arachnoid membrane separating
clot from the brain

Dura inserted into lambdoid
suture

FIGURE 2.10. CT scan with line drawings showing acute subdural haematoma, which is spread over the whole surface of the brain since the subdural space is continuous. Compare with EDH (Fig. 2.9), which is restricted by suture lines and hence biconvex in shape.

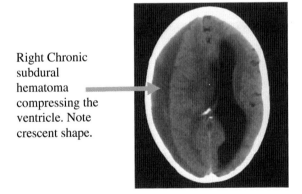

Right Chronic subdural hematoma compressing the ventricle. Note crescent shape.

FIGURE 2.11. CT scan showing right *chronic* SDH again illustrating that subdural haematomas can spread from frontal area to occipital without restriction so they tend to be shaped like a sickle or crescent with the concave surface towards the brain.

The Base of the Skull

The skull base serves as the cup that contains the brain. In doing so, it serves as the gateway for blood vessels to reach the brain and for the spinal cord to leave the skull. This 'cup' is divided into three different sections (Fig. 2.12) called anterior (pink) middle (orange) and posterior (yellow) cranial fossae. The

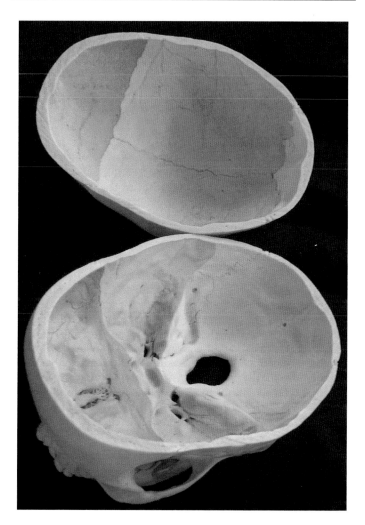

FIGURE 2.12. Interior of skull base showing anterior, middle and posterior cranial fossae.

big hole in the posterior fossa transmits the spinal cord and is called the foramen magum. The rest of the posterior fossa is filled by the cerebellum, the pons and medulla. The temporal lobe sits in the middle fossa and the frontal lobe rests in the anterior fossa.

THE 5Ss OF ANY HAEMATOMA!

What else would you consider important to note about a blood clot if you found one on a brain CT scan? STOP and write down your answer to that question before you proceed to look at the simple suggestions I have outlined as the 5Ss for easy reference.

The First S Stands for Size

In *every* CT scan, there is a scale in centimetres by each image that enables you to measure accurately the thickness of the clot and the length measured from the front to back of the clot. In addition you can count the number of slices in which the clot is visible. So by saying that the clot is about 4 cm thick and visible on 6 slices (each slice is about 0.5 cm thick or as specified) and measuring 5 cm from the front to back, you have described a clot of approximately 60 cm^3 volume ($4 \times 5 \times 3$). This may not be very informative so as you get more experienced you will be considering mostly whether a clot is immediately life threatening or not and your responsibility is to transmit that information to a neurosurgeon. The things that enable you make that judgment in addition to the size are the other four Ss, so read on!

Another practical way of conveying size is to say how many times the clot is thicker than the skull! So the size together with the other 4 Ss will give you an indication of the urgency of any clot, so let us go ahead and explore them. Note, however, that what the neurosurgeon decides to do with each of these haematomas (Fig. 2.13) will depend on the clinical condition of the patient, hence the *symptoms and signs (the neurological symptoms and signs of the patient)* are very important. The epidural haematoma was associated with a compound depressed fracture so it was operated on, and the patient with the subdural haematoma was 18 years and deeply comatose with ipsilateral dilated pupil so a decompressive craniectomy with evacuation of the subdural haematoma was carried out (Fig. 2.13). 'Although the information you get from the CT scan is the same, the neurosurgical intervention is ALWAYS determined as much by the clinical features, hence *always seek the background clinical information when looking at a brain CT scan.*'

The Second S Therefore Stands for Symptoms and Signs

By and large this is the most important part of looking at a brain CT scan because you always have to make a judgement whether

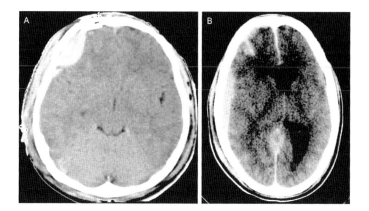

FIGURE 2.13. Example of acute epidural haematoma (A) and an acute subdural haematoma (B).

the abnormality you see is consistent with the clinical findings. Alternatively the clinical history guides you on where to look in detail on the CT scan. For instance; if the main symptom is left hemiparesis then you immediately focus on the right side of the brain. Similarly if a right-handed patient presents with speech disturbance following trauma you will look in detail at the left temporal lobe for abnormality.

However for large haematomas, even if the patient is clinically well, the blood clot is evacuated because of imminent catastrophic neurological decline, hence they should be treated as extremely urgent (see below). Perhaps the most important clinical advice to the frontline doctor with regards to emergency brain CT scan for trauma or any other reason is for you to look at the scan as soon as it is done. *This book is written to provide you a simple and easy guide on how to look at a brain CT scan and make a valid judgement for your next management action.* It does not replace a formal report from a radiologist but allows you to evaluate the CT scan and make a decision in the vast majority of cases thereby allowing you to be more efficient and improve your prioritization when multiple injuries occur. The indications for a brain CT scan in trauma are a *history* of altered level of consciousness, focal neurological deficit, skull fracture, persistent severe headache with or without vomiting and seizures following trauma to the head. The exercises at the end of this chapter will illustrate further the importance of clinical correlation in reviewing a brain CT scan but suffice it to say that large clots like the ones illustrated here (Fig. 2.14) invariably are evacuated as there is significant *shift of the brain*.

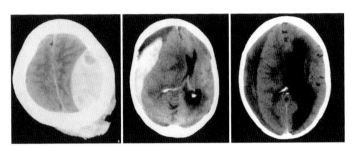

FIGURE 2.14. Large haematomas with mass effect. Emergency action required!

The Third S Stands for Shifts and Serious Consequences

The word shift implies that there is normally a boundary and indeed there are several boundaries. The midline of the brain is marked by the falx cerebri, a sheet of dura hanging down from the top of the skull (sagittal suture). As the blood clot in say Fig. 2.14 enlarges, it squashes the brain and the CSF is the first thing to be squeezed out (literally). It is very much like a sponge soaked with water. When you squeeze, the water goes out first. Similarly squeezing of the brain by a clot leads to loss of CSF from the intracranial to the lumbar cistern. This is followed by the clot pushing the brain across the midline as well as squashing it together like in Figs. 2.14 and 2.15.

The importance of these shifts is that the *pressure* on the brain (increased intracranial pressure) also prevents adequate amount of blood reaching the brain from the heart. Also if the temporal lobe is pushed over the edge of the tentorium, it compresses the third nerve giving rise to a fixed and dilated pupil on the same *side* as the clot (tentorial herniation, Fig. 2.16).

The Fourth S Stands for Side

The CT scan image normally carries with it important information such as the **patient's name, age or date of birth and the date of the scan.** But equally important it also states which side is '**left**' and '**right**'. By convention, the CT image is viewed from above with the patient supine, for instance, as if you are looking at the axial section from the head towards the feet so that the

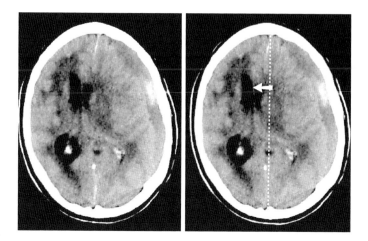

FIGURE 2.15. Chronic subdural haematoma compressing the brain and shifting the midline from the white line to the arrow tip.

right side of the brain appears on the viewer's left and the left brain appears on the viewer's right on the screen. However, as Fig. 2.17 shows the image can be horizontally flipped electronically or manually misplaced in the x-ray viewing box and unless you check the labelling 'religiously', you risk misleading yourself about the side.

Note that Fig. 2.18 is exactly the same as Fig. 2.17 except that I removed the labels from Fig. 2.17. So without looking at the labels, the mistake in Fig. 2.17 cannot be corrected. 'Finally CT films are only images and clearly can be corrupted or be subject to any number of errors. *As a result, an opinion on the CT scan is meaningless unless correlated with the patient's clinical history and signs.* Nowhere is that assertion any more true than with regard to the side of the lesion.'

The 5th S stands for the Site of the Haematoma

The site of a clot is very important because haematomas inside the brain are classified (and named by their location). Just like your name is your identity, where a clot is located defines the identity of that clot. We saw earlier that epidural and subdural haematomas are so named because of their relationship to the dura. The second dimension in considering *site* is the part of the brain or the skull the clot is related to. For instance, Fig. 2.19A

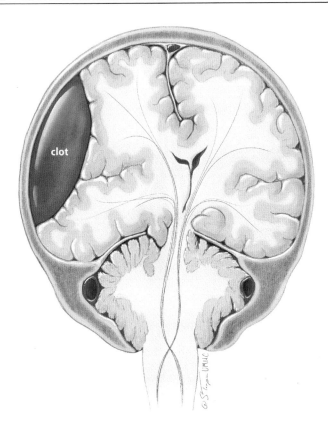

FIGURE 2.16. Schematic diagram showing tentorial herniation. (Note that this finding is an extreme emergency requiring immediate neurosurgical intervention. *'In this situation a double strength of adrenaline is required – NOT for the patient but for the frontline doctor to move fast!)'*

is called a small left frontal epidural haematoma because it is an epidural haematoma located between the frontal bone and the left frontal lobe of the brain. Similarly Fig. 2.19B will be called a large right frontal and temporal subdural haematoma because it is a subdural clot located both in the frontal and temporal areas. You will notice two things. First is that the subdural haematomas spread across two areas of the cranium freely because there are no barriers (sutures) restricting it like you find with the epidural haematoma, which is convex and confined to under the frontal

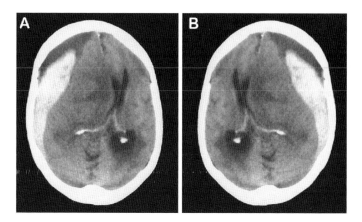

FIGURE 2.17A and B. On which side of the brain is this clot? It is so easy to inadvertently flip the CT films or the convention adopted may be different from what you are used to; so ALWAYS CHECK THE LABELLING OF LEFT AND RIGHT! See Fig. 2.18.

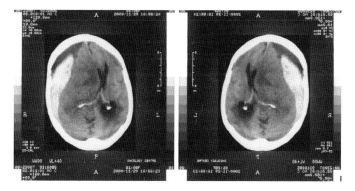

FIGURE 2.18. Showing the ease with which error can occur if the side labels are not checked ALWAYS!

bone alone due to the restricting effect of the dura. The second thing is that in naming these haematomas, I have been careful to mention the sides just like we learnt above. Can you notice any other things about Fig. 2.19B that are important? See below.

The following phrases about *site* may be clarified at this time: ***intracranial haemorrhage or haematoma*** (cranium = skull) refers to haemorrhage anywhere within the skull, of any cause. Therefore epidural haematoma, subdural haematoma and

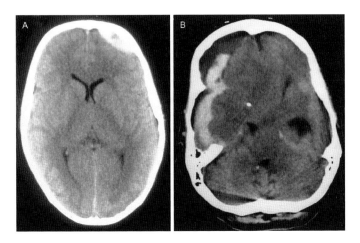

FIGURE 2.19. A and B showing a small left frontal acute epidural haematoma and a large right frontal and temporal acute subdural haematoma. Can you comment on the acute subdural haematoma with regards to size, shift and severe consequences?

subarachnoid haemorrhage and intracerebral haematoma are all different types of *intracranial haemorrhage* distinguished only by the layer (depth in the brain) in which the blood clot forms. Note that *intracerebral haematomas* are clots located entirely within the substance of the brain or the larger part of it is in the substance of the brain but may track into the ventricles or into the subdural space. Contusions are small intracerebral haemorrhages that often occur in areas where the brain comes in contact with the very rough floor of the skull like the floor of the frontal lobe (Fig. 2.21A) and the temporal lobe. They also occur in deeper brain structures from shear injury (Fig. 2.20) and larger contusions form intracerebral haematomas (Figs. 2.2 and 2.6).

Clots are defined by:

- Size
- Symptoms and signs
- Shifts
- Side
- site

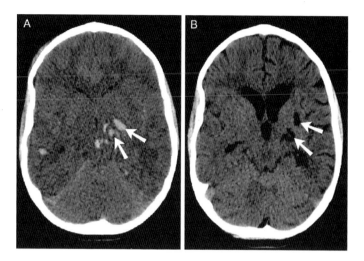

FIGURE 2.20. CT scan showing early- and late-appearance left basal ganglia and external capsule contusions. Note the right temporal contusion also in the early scan. In the late scan, the contusion has resolved leaving behind a low-density cavity.

Although haematomas have been emphasized here, by far the more common abnormality seen on brain CT scan following trauma is swelling from diffuse axonal injury. Figure 2.21 shows two children – one with a skull fracture and brain contusions but not diffuse swelling (images A, B and C) and the other with diffuse axonal injury (images D, E and F). The skull fracture child made a complete recovery but the diffuse axonal injury was fatal. Thus in Fig. 2.21A, B and C despite the significant skull fracture, brain swelling is minimal and the third ventricle is clearly visible. The clear visualization of the third ventricle and the basal cisterns is usually presumptive evidence that there *may not be* severe diffuse brain swelling. However, complete lack of visualization of the third ventricle and basal cisterns is indicative of severe swelling as in Fig. 2.21F. Also if you compare Fig. 2.21D and E, which are scans done 3 days apart on the same child, it is obvious that the 4th ventricle is no longer visible in Fig. 2.21E due to swelling. There is also loss of grey white differentiation in the image series Fig. 2.21D, E and F. *'Note that A and B of Fig. 2.21 are the same slice of CT scan but in Fig. 2.21B, the window level has been set to show bony anomalies clearly. This is called the bone window, and*

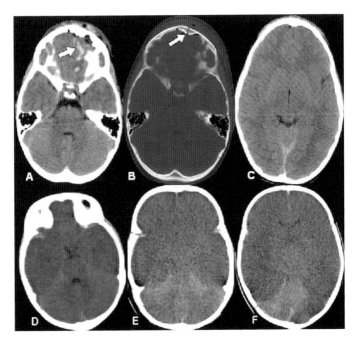

FIGURE 2.21. Examples of different traumatic lesions: A, B and C are CT scans from a 6-year-old with left frontal fracture and contusions from a motor vehicle collision. Images D, E and F are from a *different* child with shaken baby syndrome with diffuse axonal injury. A = shows left frontal contusion (white arrow); B = the same scan as A but in the bone window showing left frontal skull fracture (white arrow), which is difficult to see on the normal window in A; C = illustrates the ready visualization of the third ventricle signifying the absence of diffuse swelling; D and E are from the child with shaken baby syndrome with the scans done three days apart showing the absence of the 4th ventricle in E due to swelling and the loss of grey white differentiation in F.

it is essential for seeing linear fractures especially at the base of the skull.'

To summarize, clots over the motor cortex (posterior frontal) will cause hemiparesis on the contralateral (opposite) side. Also commonly left temporal contusions and haematomas will present with dysphasia because in the majority of right-handed people the left temporal lobe is responsible for speech. So you can see that the site of a clot is very important. Hence I encourage you to briefly look up Fig. 1.20 again so that you are familiar with the parts of the brain and their function.

The red flags in Fig. 2.19B that I expected you to identify were the subfalcine herniation, the significant midline shift to the left and contralateral hydrocephalus indicated by the enlarged temporal horn. All these features come to one conclusion: Emergency action required!

'In other words, even if the patient appears stable and has a clot like the one in Fig. 2.19B with compression of the brain and midline shift, they are on a dangerous and sloppy edge so emergency action is required. And if they are comatose with a scan like that then it constitutes an ***extreme emergency!***'

Chapter 3
Brain Haemorrhage and Infarction – Stroke

SUBARACHNOID HAEMORRHAGE

Bleeding into the subarachnoid space is called subarachnoid haemorrhage to distinguish it from bleeding into the substance of the brain proper, which is called intracerebral haemorrhage or intracerebral haematoma. The distinction is important because spontaneous subarachnoid haemorrhage is most frequently caused by aneurysm rupture, which is fatal in one third of cases. Second haemorrhages carry even a higher fatality rate, hence it is imperative to detect any subarachnoid haemorrhage and treat the underlying aneurysm (Fig. 3.1). Aneurysms are blowouts of the major arteries as they enter the base of the brain close to the skull base, especially at arterial bifurcations.

The basic concept to start from is that the subarachnoid spaces in the brain are practically continuous spreading from left to right across the midline and from the base of the skull to the top (Fig. 3.2). The second concept to appreciate is that the main blood vessels in the brain *travel* in the subarachnoid space, hence when an aneurysm ruptures, it bleeds into the subarachnoid space where there is very little to tamponade the bleed and stop it early! It also explains why bleeding easily spreads from left to right and vice versa.

The majority of aneurysms occur around the circle of Willis, hence aneurysmal subarachnoid haemorrhage tends to appear mainly in the basal cisterns and sylvian fissure on CT scan, and thankfully most cases are obvious as in Fig. 3.3.

U. Igbaseimokumo, *Brain CT Scans in Clinical Practice*,
DOI 10.1007/b98343_3, © Springer-Verlag London Limited 2009

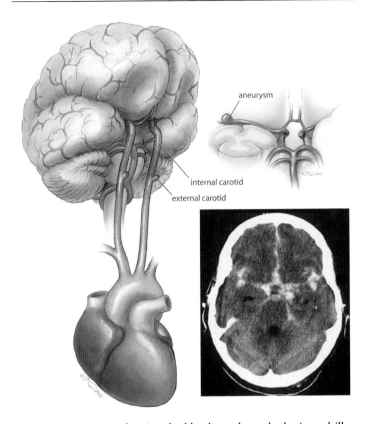

FIGURE 3.1. Drawing showing the blood supply to the brain and illustrating an aneurysm in the middle cerebral artery. A CT scan showing widespread SAH from such an aneurysm is also given. Compare with Fig. 3.2, an MRI showing how the vessels travel in the subarachnoid space, and note that the subarachnoid space is continuous from right to left.

If all SAH were as obvious as the images in Fig. 3.3 then this chapter would be very short! Not infrequently the amount of blood maybe so small that the inexperienced physician could miss subtle features of SAH on the CT scan, hence a systematic approach is required to examine a CT scan for clues.

It is important however to emphasize that the mere absence of visible blood on CT scan *does not exclude SAH*, but a lumbar

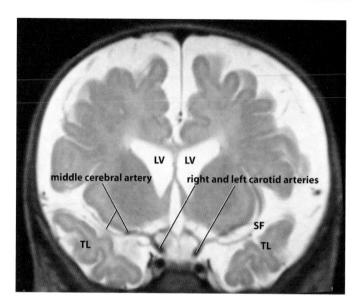

FIGURE 3.2. Coronal MRI at the level of the sylvian fissure (SF) show-ing the free communication of the subarachnoid space from the base of the skull to the convexity on either side and how the main blood vessels travel in the subarachnoid space. The carotid arteries divide into anterior cerebral and middle cerebral arteries. The left and right anterior cerebral arteries are linked by the anterior communicating artery and two pos-terior cerebral arteries are linked to each carotid via the left and right posterior communicating arteries, thus making up the circle of Willis – the arterial ring that supplies blood to the brain. (LV = lateral ventricle; SF = Sylvian fissure; TL = Temporal lobes).

puncture is required in patients with a history suggestive of SAH who appear not to have visible blood on the CT scan.

Figure 3.4 shows different degrees of obviousness of SAH, but the most important lesson is to note the usual locations when blood is obvious so that when SAH is not obvious, the usual locations can be *scrutinized* with a magnifying glass for any suspicious densities or other clue of SAH! With this background, we can now consider the thought process involved in evaluating a *patient*'s CT scan for SAH in the emergency room or anywhere for that matter. The following points are key to pre-venting error.

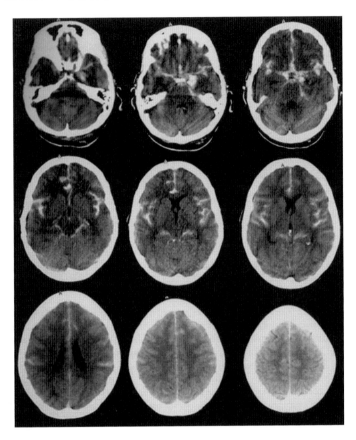

FIGURE 3.3. Non-contrast CT scan showing widespread SAH. Note the symmetrical outline of the left and right sylvian fissures and how the blood has outlined all the basal CSF spaces.

First Clue in SAH Is the Clinical History

The first universally agreed principle is that when it comes to SAH, the history is the key factor in determining the doctor's course of action or investigation of the patient. Nowhere else is a good history as vital in the evaluation of a neurological patient as in SAH. Let us briefly examine the history as it applies to the brain CT scan interpretation. The sensitivity of a CT scan in picking up SAH is 95% within the first twenty-four hours and this drops to 84% after three days and 50% at the end of a week. ***It is therefore obvious that the CT appearances of SAH change***

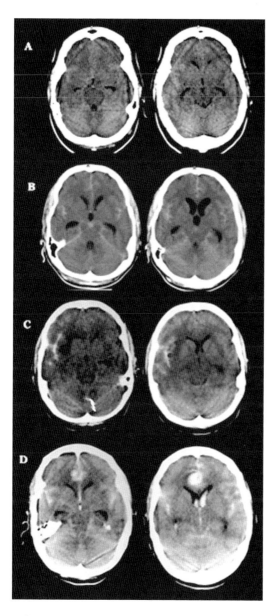

FIGURE 3.4. (continued)

with time so a clear history of the time of onset of symptoms is important in your interpretation of the CT findings. The typical history is of sudden onset severe headache with or without loss of consciousness, often characterized as the worst-ever headache the patient has experienced. As mentioned earlier, if the CT scan is negative, then a lumbar puncture is required to exclude SAH and in cases with a typical history a neurosurgeon should be consulted to discuss the final disposal of the patient as angiography may still be required in highly selected cases even if the CT and lumbar puncture are inconclusive of SAH!

"Listen to the history with intent" and "Look at the CT scan with intent" *to find blood.*

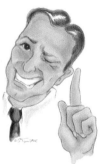

The following pages
will assist you
to learn where to focus
and
what to look for
on the CT scan
if SAH is suspected!

FIGURE 3.4. (continued) Different degrees of obviousness of SAH are shown: (A) The hyperdensity in the interhemispheric and right sylvian fissure and ambient cisterns along with early hydrocephalus make the diagnosis of SAH pretty secure. (B) The bilateral sylvian and interhemispheric blood (hyperdensities) is fairly obvious and the hydrocephalus is now clear cut with a rounded third ventricle and dilated temporal horns. (C) Here consideration of the right and left sylvian fissures shows obvious blood in the right sylvian fissure. The important point however is that the left sylvian fissure is almost not visualized but it is obviously present! So in a suspected case of SAH, the sylvian fissure should be inspected in detail with a magnifying glass knowing that if blood were present it would perhaps take the shapes shown in Fig. 3.4B and C. (D) Shows a haematoma in the interhemispheric fissure along with intraventricular blood and bilateral sylvian fissure blood. SAH is obvious here.

Where to Look for SAH – Usual Locations

The obvious cases of SAH like in Fig. 3.3 will pose little problem to even the most busy frontline doctor. However, a systematic approach and more **TIME** are required to identify less obvious cases and to determine early complications including hydrocephalus, infarction, giant aneurysms and haematomas, which maybe associated with SAH.

The Interhemispheric Fissure

The interhemispheric fissure is the home of the anterior communicating artery and anterior cerebral artery aneurysms, the commonest site of aneurysms. Subarachnoid haemorrhage here is characterized by interheimispheric blood or haematoma and not infrequently it ruptures into the ventricle as in Fig. 3.5C.

The Sylvian Fissures

The sylvian fissures are home to middle cerebral artery aneurysms. It is important to note that the sylvian fissures communicate freely with the central sulcus and other sulci that run to the convexity of the brain as shown by the blood in Fig. 3.6 (compare with Fig. 3.2). Occasionally the blood in the basal part is washed off by the CSF turnover, leaving a streak of blood in

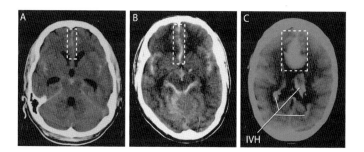

FIGURE 3.5. Non-contrast axial CT scans showing different amounts of blood visible in the interhemispheric fissure (dotted boxes). The idea is to look carefully in this location on all the slices with one intention only – to find blood if present! Note carefully that the quality of the CT scan can vary widely even from the same machine due to differences in brightness of the images as produced for you by the radiographer. The intraventricular haemorrhage (IVH) in image (C) is obvious but the overall quality of this image is poor. *'If the image quality is unsatisfactory for any reason, then be sure to have a neuroradiologist review the films or have the radiographer repeat them!'*

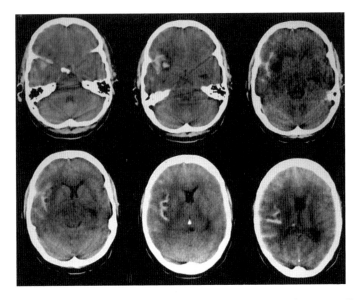

FIGURE 3.6. Non-contrast CT scan showing right sylvian fissure small haematoma and subarachnoid blood. *'The important point is that the subarachnoid spaces are barely visible on the opposite side.'* In less obvious cases, it is the areas corresponding to where the blood is seen on the right that are scrutinized for any evidence of blood. Can you try finding the CSF spaces on the left corresponding to the spaces where the blood is seen on the right?

the convexity sulci alone. This should be appreciated as possibly coming from an aneurysm.

The Ambient Cisterns

The ambient cisterns surround the midbrain and communicate with the interpeduncular fossa where the circle of Willis is located. Bleeding into this space could come from several places and is easily recognized by the *'loss'* of the dark CSF density around the midbrain. So that even if they (the ambient cisterns which are normally hypodense) were to appear isodense with brain, then a focused scrutiny is required to look for other evidence of SAH. Of course if the presence of blood is as obvious as the case in Fig. 3.7, the diagnosis is easy.

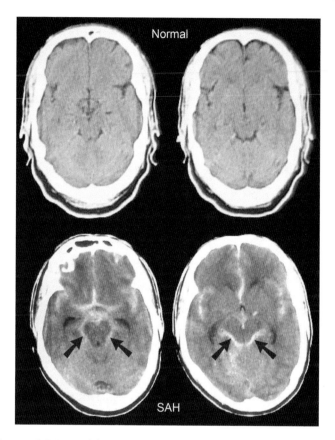

FIGURE 3.7. Normal brain CT scan with normal ambient cisterns with hypodense CSF (above pair) and what they look like in the presence of subarachnoid haemorrhage (black arrows) in the image pair below. Note that there is widespread blood in the other CSF spaces as well (interhemispheric, sylvian fissure and the suprasellar cisterns).

Prepontine Cisterns

The prepontine cistern is a very important location to scrutinize for SAH because basilar tip aneurysms make their home here and hyperdense blood from SAH could be easily obscured by the surrounding bone, which forms the anterior boundary of this space (Figs. 3.8 and 3.9).

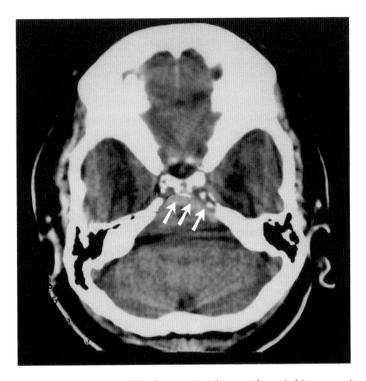

FIGURE 3.8. Clear example of prepontine haemorrhage (white arrows). However, there are frequent artefacts in the posterior fossa slices of the CT scan making the detection of such a lesion in less obvious cases difficult, hence there is the need for focused scrutiny of this location.

Associated Features or Complications: The H.I.G.H of SAH
HIGH stands for *H*ydrocephalus, *I*nfarction, *G*iant aneurysms and *H*aematoma.

Hydrocephalus as a Subtle Sign of SAH
Hydrocephalus (often transient) is a frequent accompaniment of SAH. In mild or early hydrocephalus, the patient often gives a typical history of sudden onset severe headache, a day or more before presentation to hospital. The brain CT scan may show only early hydrocephalus characterized by dilatation of the temporal horns of the lateral ventricles. This should be taken as a strong clue of recent SAH because in the normal brain scan (Fig. 3.10) the temporal horns are usually not visible or barely

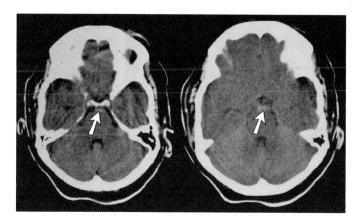

FIGURE 3.9. Shows the CT scan of a 51-year-old hypertensive and diabetic lady with sudden onset severe headache described as the worst headache of her life. She was alert but had neck stiffness and mild photophobia. The small haemorrhage in front of the pons could easily be overlooked unless this area is scrutinized. That it is not an artefact is confirmed by tracing its continuity on contiguous slices. *'It is far safer to err on the cautious side and have a more experienced person review the films should you see these appearances on only one slice or suspect they are artefacts!'*

seen on focused search. But in early hydrocephalus as may occur following SAH, the temporal horns become clearly visible or comparable in size to the frontal horns as seen in Fig. 3.10. In more severe cases, the hydrocephalus is obvious with a rounded third ventricle (instead of being slit like) and the temporal horns are obviously dilated (Fig. 3.10). Thus a suggestive clinical history plus the finding of early hydrocephalus on the CT scan is presumptive evidence of SAH and requires further review of the images by a neuroradiologist or further investigation including a lumbar puncture. When blood is evident as in Fig. 3.6 (above), the diagnosis is certain and the next investigation is angiography to locate the source of the subarachnoid haemorrhage (Fig. 3.15 below).

Hydrocephalus as an Acute Emergency
Not infrequently hydrocephalus is catastrophic and becomes the immediate cause of death, hence the survival of those who get to the CT scanner depends on the immediate appreciation of the CT appearances and quick response of the frontline doctor. In this situation, the patient usually suddenly lapses into deep coma

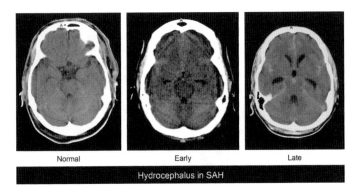

Normal   Early   Late

Hydrocephalus in SAH

FIGURE 3.10. Axial non-contrast CT scans showing normal ventricles and early hydrocephalus in a 48-year-old female school teacher who gave a 24-h history of sudden severe headache. She had neck stiffness and had vomited twice. The early hydrocephalus is much more easily visible than the increased hyperdensity in the right sylvian fissure and interhemispheric fissure and right ambient cisterns. In the more severe and late case of hydrocephalus following SAH, the temporal horns are larger and the third ventricle is rounded with obvious residual SAH visible in the usual locations bilaterally. Can you name all the spaces containing blood, considering left and right separately?

requiring respiratory support with clinical evidence of brain stem compromise (coning). The CT scan shows blood filling and dilating the ventricular system (all 4 ventricles) as well as widespread subarachnoid haemorrhage in the usual locations (Fig. 3.11). It is particularly important to transmit this information to the neurosurgeon as brain-specific intervention such as external ventricular drain may be life saving and may have to be integrated into the early resuscitative effort, following the ABCs of resuscitation.

Infarction
Low densities in the brain parenchyma associated with a recent ($\geq$3–10 days) history of SAH when present implies established or imminent infarction or oedema of the brain (Fig. 3.12). It often occurs following widespread SAH and unlike ischemic stroke with clear margins (see below), the hypodensities in SAH tend to cross vascular boundaries and be more pronounced in the watershed areas, i.e. the boundary areas between the blood supply of the anterior cerebral and middle cerebral arteries. This complication which represents vasospasm with ischemia usually

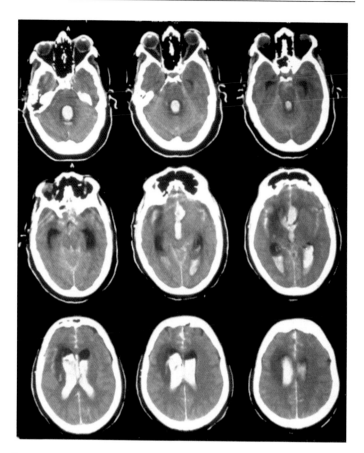

FIGURE 3.11. Non-contrast brain CT scan showing massive intraventricular haemorrhage with hydrocephalus as well as widespread subarachnoid haemorrhage. The patient was aged 45 years and suddenly slumped on top of his wife during intercourse.

occurs after the third day, and hence it may be seen in inpatients or patients transferred from other hospitals or in patients who present late especially in parts of the world where CT scans are not readily available.

Giant Aneurysms

Giant or large aneurysms may be visible on brain CT scan. They exert a lot of mass effect and may precipitate hydrocephalus. The differential diagnosis to consider is a tumour. Aneurysms

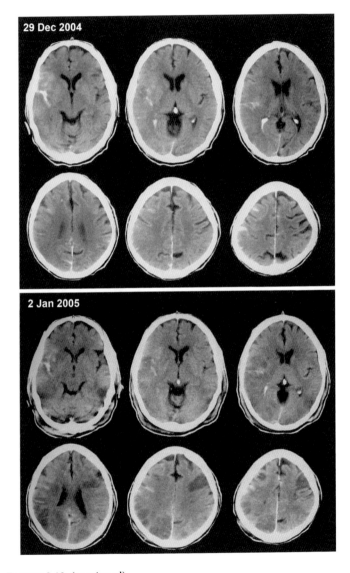

FIGURE 3.12. (continued)

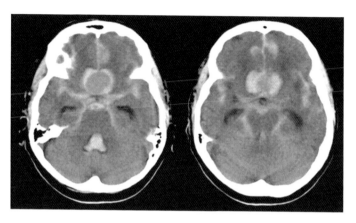

FIGURE 3.13. Brain CT scan showing a giant anterior communicating artery aneurysm. Note the widespread SAH and hydrocephalus. The outline of the aneurysm is enhanced by the blood surrounding the wall in the interhemispheric fissure.

generally have a more smooth and rounded outline compared to tumours and are often located in the areas where aneurysms are usually found – the suprasellar cistern and the sylvian fissures. In addition, SAH associated with tumours like gliomas, meningioma or pituitary tumors for example, is a very rare occurrence. Therefore, a mass lesion like in Fig. 3.13 in association with SAH equals a large aneurysm until proven otherwise and you should act quickly.

FIGURE 3.12. (continued) Initial and follow-up CT scans of a 70-year-old male showing hypodense lesions consistent with watershed infarcts from SAH. He was noticed to have fallen down clutching his head. This case also illustrates the important clinical situation when trauma follows the collapse from SAH. It becomes imperative to determine if the SAH was primary or secondary to trauma. Although a large volume of blood in the basal cisterns often suggests primary (aneurysmal SAH) and blood over the convexity associated with fractures may point to trauma, the distinction may not be clear cut.

Haematoma

Subarachnoid haemorrhage associated with intracerebral haematoma also signifies large volume of haemorrhage and the location is often in the temporal lobe (middle cerebral artery aneurysm) or the frontal lobes – interhemispheric haematoma from anterior communicating artery aneurysm. The typical appearance consists of subarachnoid haemorrhage in the usual locations associated with a large hyperdense clot inside the brain proper. The important differential diagnosis here is hypertensive intracerebral haemorrhage, which can be distinguished from aneurysmal haemorrhage with haematoma by the classic basal ganglia location of the former (see below) as well as the lack of a significant SAH. The CT appearances of the two types of lesions may occasionally be indistinguishable, but from a practical point of view, both require review by a neurosurgeon and or a neuroradiologist but the accurate description of the appearances to a neurosurgeon may be life saving (Fig. 3.14).

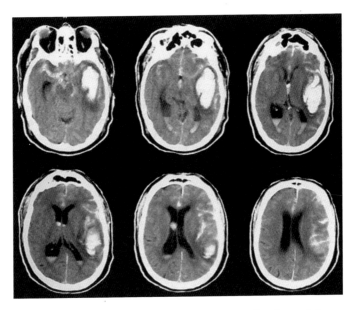

FIGURE 3.14. Non-contrast axial CT brain scan showing a left temporal haematoma and widespread subarachnoid haemorrhage. Can you identify all the CSF spaces where blood is visible? At least five named spaces are filled with blood – counting left and right separately!

TABLE 3.1. Key steps in looking for SAH

1. Compare left and right
2. Look for SAH in the sulci, remember blood will settle into the
sulci not on the gyri.
3. Look in the usual locations – sylvian fissure, interhemispheric
fissure, basal and prepontine cisterns.
4. Look for associated features like hydrocephalus, infarction,
giant aneurysms and haematoma.
5. Above ALL – remember the clinical history is your best clue!

Epilogue on CT Scan for SAH

Table 3.1 shows the basic approach to identifying SAH on a CT scan. The gold standard for detecting aneurysms at present is digital subtraction angiography (Fig. 3.15), so the principal question at stake if a clinically well patient complains of sudden severe headache suggestive of SAH but the CT scan does not show blood is 'should they have an angiogram or not?' If the CT scan is negative, a lumbar puncture is widely accepted as ruling out SAH if performed properly. The significant number of traumatic taps and the lack of universally agreed criteria for measuring xanthochromia raise doubt on the use of this test as gold standard. In any event, the issue is to balance the risks (and perhaps cost) of angiography against the morbidity of fearing the worst with every subsequent headache, so the patient's choice may eventually drive clinical practice. Hence, the advent of CT angiography may well see a change in practice such that a positive SAH immediately proceeds to CT angiography. And the question remains open as to what will happen with the CT negative patient – a CT angiogram or a lumbar puncture? A lumbar puncture may continue to be necessary to confirm if an aneurysm has actually bled as the natural history of incidental aneurysm is different from that of a previously ruptured aneurysm.

SPONTANEOUS INTRACEREBRAL HAEMATOMA

Spontaneous intracerebral haemorrhage occurs inside the brain substance proper (for instance inside the parenchyma of the brain) as opposed to subarachnoid haemorrhage, which bleeds into the subarachnoid space. It is called spontaneous to distinguish it from traumatic intracerebral haematoma. It is perhaps helpful to learn that intracerebral haematoma also has special locations which together with the etiology gives it a unique

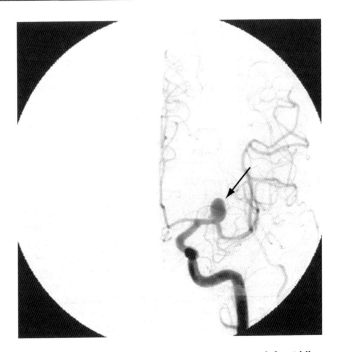

FIGURE 3.15. Digital subtraction angiogram showing a left middle cerebral artery aneurysm (arrow).

identity. Whereas rebleed is the principal concern in the majority of cases of subarachnoid haemorrhage, the principal concern in intracerebral haematoma is the mass effect and functional damage. Whereas the good grade SAH patient may expect to live a normal life with appropriate successful treatment, the patient with a small internal capsule haemorrhage may be hemiplegic for life with little recourse to surgery. While clinically significant intracerebral haematomas are obvious on the CT scan, subarachnoid haemorrhage may be difficult to detect, yet the underlying aneurysm remains lethal should it bleed again. In addition, most patients with significant intracerebral haematoma except few polar haemorrhages will have significant findings on neurological examination, but up to 50% of patients with SAH show no neurologic finding except the headache that brought them to the emergency care physician! Therefore in this chapter, the

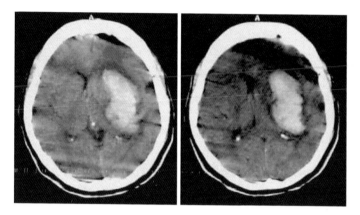

FIGURE 3.16. Non-contrast axial CT scan of a 31-year-old male with sudden right hemiplegia and altered level of consciousness, showing a large left basal ganglia/internal capsular haemorrhage. Note the movement artefacts as the patient was restless and not fully co-operative. The lesion is obvious in spite of the artefacts and of course the quality of the CT image may vary from place to place depending on resources, but the rule of thumb is that 'only the best image is good enough for interpretation in order not to miss a small abnormality'!

emphasis has been on detection of SAH without trivializing the importance of intracerebral haematomas (Fig. 3.16).

Usual Locations and Aetiology

Spontaneous intracerebral haematoma is often the result of uncontrolled hypertension or amyloid angiopathy. The lenticulostriate vessels (Fig. 3.17) arise from the middle cerebral artery bringing relatively high hydrostatic pressure from the carotid to the internal capsule, basal ganglia and thalamus. These areas are therefore prone to hypertensive haemorrhage and are the usual locations although a large haemorrhage could rupture into the ventricles (Fig. 3.18) and confuse the beginner in neuroradiology or emergency medicine.

Spontaneous intracerebral haematomas may be obvious on the scan, but telling someone else on the phone or in written form requires a clear description of the size and location of the clot. Therefore, a basic understanding of few key structures in the brain (Fig. 3.19) is essential to understanding the importance of an intracerebral haematoma.

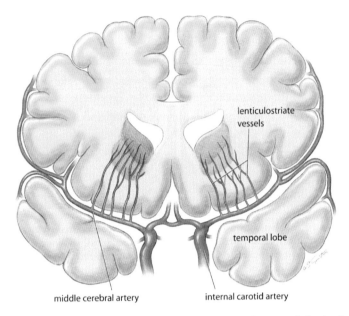

FIGURE 3.17. Drawing of the cerebral vessels with part of the brain removed to show the lenticulostriate vessels that are responsible for haemorrhage in hypertension (and infarction in ischemic stroke [see below]).

Basic CT Scan Internal Landmarks

The anatomy of the brain can be viewed simplistically as a mushroom or umbrella in which the stem is formed by the brain stem and the cerebral hemispheres represent the cap of the umbrella. The brain stem consists of the medulla oblongata (no. 1 in Fig. 3.19), pons (no. 2 in Fig. 3.19) and the midbrain (no. 3 in Fig. 3.19). The pons is easily identified as the quadrangular mass in front of the fourth ventricle often with the basilar artery visible in front of it (images D and E in Fig. 3.19). Thus as soon as you identify the fourth ventricle, the pons is in front and the medulla is below the pons and the midbrain above it. The lazy 'V' facing laterally (Fig. 3.19H) marks the position of the internal capsule, a key structure in this part of the brain. The caudate nucleus (no. 5 in Fig. 3.19) and the thalamus (no. 4 in Fig. 3.19) are medial to the internal capsule whereas the remainder of the basal ganglia – the lentiform nucleus (no. 6 in Fig. 3.19) is lateral to the internal capsule, for instance

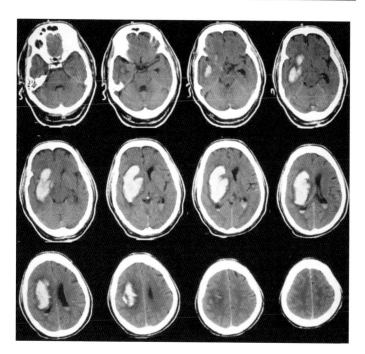

FIGURE 3.18. Non-contrast CT scan of a 60-year-old male who developed sudden left hemiplegia and headache but was alert and orientated. It shows a large left internal capsular haemorrhage, which has ruptured into the ventricles. Note that in spite of the size of the intracerebral haematoma, there is very little SAH. Compare with Fig. 3.14, which is aneurysmal SAH with an intracerebral haematoma.

contained in the 'V'. Thus close scrutiny of Fig. 3.18 will show that the haematoma started in the lentiform nucleus and ruptured into the ventricles. The caudate nucleus, thalamus, internal capsule and the lentiform nucleus represent the important areas supplied by the lenticulostriate arteries illustrated in Fig. 3.17, hence this area is the typical location of hypertensive haemorrhage (Fig. 3.18). Similarly, ischemic stroke affects the same areas frequently.

As I mentioned in Chapter 1, understanding the CSF spaces in the brain CT scan is key to interpreting a CT scan. Thus the fourth ventricle is an important landmark: the pons is in front of it and behind the fourth ventricle is the *cerebellum* (see Chapter 1). Haemorrhage into the cerebellum (Fig. 3.20) or pons (if large

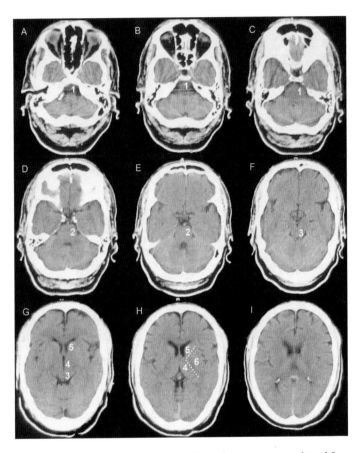

FIGURE 3.19. Non-contrast CT scan with vital structures numbered from 1 to 5 and the individual slices are labelled from A to I. Can you identify each of the numbered structures? See text for answers.

enough) may compress the fourth ventricle or rupture into the fourth ventricle leading to hydrocephalus. Therefore, if you see a haemorrhage (blood clot) in the cerebellum or pons, you must immediately ask yourself the question, is there hydrocephalus (see Chapter 4). Thus haemorrhages here (cerebellum) are very important not only because of the functional loss but also because of the risk of hydrocephalus!

Haemorrhages in the cerebral hemispheres could arise from several causes including hypertension, amyloid angiopathy and

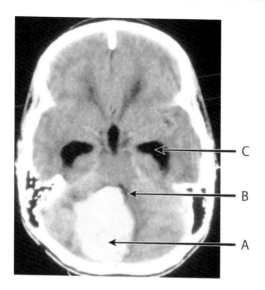

FIGURE 3.20. A non-contrast CT scan showing a large cerebellar haematoma (A) causing almost complete compression of the fourth ventricle (B) with obvious hydrocephalus seen in the dilated temporal horns (C).

arteriovenous malformations. Of these the AVMs are very important because of the risk of recurrent haemorrhage and their propensity to occur in the young patient. The clot often appears close to the brain surface (Fig. 3.21A) and there may be associated subarachnoid haemorrhage. *'It is obvious that the site and size of an intracerebral haematoma are important in determining the clinical effects of an intracerebral haematoma and that brain shifts portend catastrophic decline in clinical condition.'* Of course it goes without saying that the side of the hemisphere, left or right, is important and although the shape may not tell the beginner much, tumoral haemorrhages tend to give a clue in their shape (Fig. 3.22). *'Thus the five Ss (site, size, shifts, side and shape) will as described for traumatic haematoma also help you describe a spontaneous haematoma adequately.'*

Although haemorrhage into a tumour is far less common, the CT scan may show a double density different (white arrow in Fig. 3.23) from the haematoma and also the presence of oedema (low density) around the clot. *'Whereas these are not*

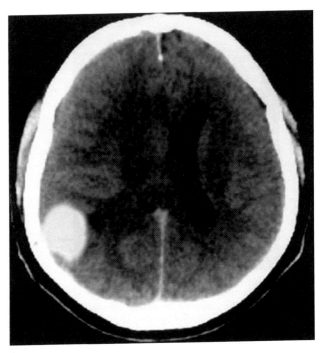

FIGURE 3.21. Non-contrast CT scan showing right parietal intracerebral haematoma secondary to an AVM. Note the surface location and the swelling in the underlying hemisphere.

pathognomonic features of tumour haemorrhage, they should point to further scrutiny of the scan.'

ISCHEMIC STROKE (CEREBRAL INFARCTION)

It is convenient to start by revising Fig. 3.17, especially the lenticulostriate vessels which supply the areas labelled nos 4, 5 and 6 in Fig. 3.19. This area is commonly involved in CVA be it hemorrhagic or thromboembolic. *'The key principle behind successful use of the CT scan in dealing with ischemic stroke is KNOWING WHERE TO LOOK! AND WHAT TO LOOK FOR! And WHEN TO LOOK!'*

Ischemic stroke will show very little signs on the CT scan within the first 2–3 h of the ictus (event) (Fig. 3.24), depending on

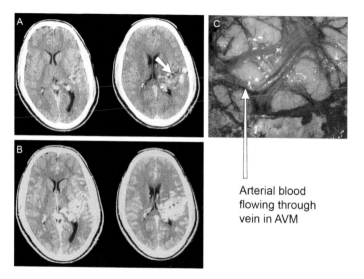

Arterial blood
flowing through
vein in AVM

FIGURE 3.22. Composite picture of a CT scan of an unruptured AVM [pre-contrast (A) and post contrast (B)] with an operative photograph showing arterialized veins and the junction of venous and arterial blood. Very cool picture!

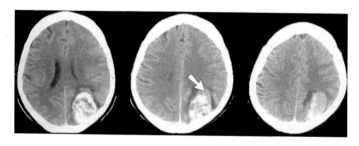

FIGURE 3.23. Non-contrast CT scan showing left parietal intracerebral haemorrhage into a tumour. Note the different density (white arrow) and the surrounding low density which represents oedema.

the area involved and the presence or absence of anastomotic collaterals and the quality of the CT scan used. *'The golden rule with stroke as with most of emergency neurosurgery or neurology is that, the clinical symptoms reign supreme.'* Therefore, for the patient in Fig. 3.24 with a right hemiplegia, the conclusion following that first CT scan is that it is too early to see obvious changes on the CT

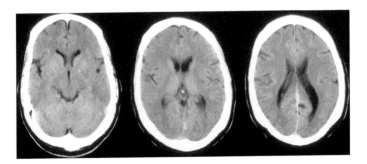

FIGURE 3.24. Non-contrast CT scan of a 61-year-old male with sudden onset right hemiplegia two and a half hours prior to the CT scan. He is diabetic and hypertensive. *'Given the history most experienced radiologists will identify the subtle differences but it may seem completely normal to a beginner. The CT findings are often only as important as the question it was intended to answer! What was the clinical question in requesting a CT scan here?'*

scan, and so a follow-up imaging is needed and the patient gets referred to a neurologist or stroke physician promptly. It should not be seen as a normal scan and the patient's treatment delayed *'as a consequence of lack of pace.'* In fact, it is a common reason in many centres to carry out the emergency CT scan in thrombotic CVA simply to confirm the absence of a mature infarct or haemorrhage prior to anticoagulation or thrombolysis. What follows therefore is one approach to describing a thromboembolic CVA bearing in mind the time-dependent nature of the CT appearances (Fig. 3.25).

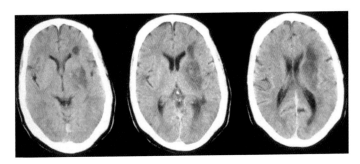

FIGURE 3.25. Non-contrast CT scan of the same patient as in Fig. 3.24 showing the now obvious left basal ganglia infarct (low density).

Ischemic stroke can be described with the acronym THOSE to signify the major events occurring.

T~ Stands for the Territory – the Vascular Territory
Because there is very little collateral circulation in the brain, thrombosis in distal arteries often leads to infarction in the area supplied by that artery. This leads to well-demarcated zones of infarction as in Fig. 3.25 that are characteristic of the supplying vessel (lenticulostriate vessels). Other common examples include the middle cerebral artery (Fig. 3.26) and the anterior cerebral artery territories.

H~ Stands for Hypodensity
The basic appearance of an infarct on CT scan is a hypo-dense lesion often with clear margins. However, as seen between Figs. 3.25 and 3.26, the hypodensity does take up to 6–8 h to appear and a clear margin such as is illustrated in Fig. 3.26 may not be obvious for days. Of course with the latest generation of CT scan machines, perfusion CT scan will invariably show up the ischemic focus well before the appearance of low density on conventional CT. Figure 3.27 shows a middle cerebral artery infarct

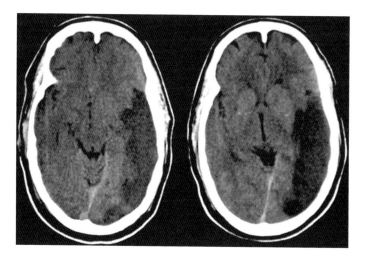

FIGURE 3.26. CT scan showing low density from left middle cerebral artery posterior division infarct.

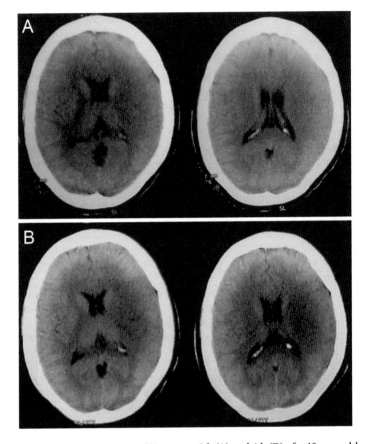

FIGURE 3.27. Non-contrast CT scans at 3 h (A) and 6 h (B) of a 40-year-old lady who presented with acute onset hemiplegia while cooking dinner in the kitchen. Can you tell which side has the low density? Do not forget the principles of comparing left and right focusing on the 'usual suspect' areas for infarction.

at 3 and 6 h after the ictus. Can you convince yourself about the low density?

O~ Stands for Oedema

The O represents a vital conceptual link between the H and the S. The hypodensity seen on CT scan actually represents *oedema* – cytotoxic oedema – that starts promptly following the occlusion

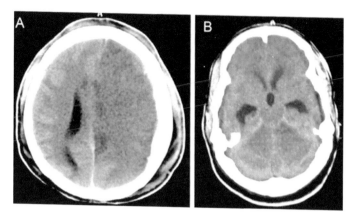

FIGURE 3.28. Non-contrast brain CT showing a massive left internal carotid territory infarct with swelling and midline shift (A) and an acute cerebellar infarct with hydrocephalus (B).

of the artery. The oedema leads to swelling of the cells with consequent sulcal effacement and brain shift.

S~Stands for Swelling and Shifts
Brain shifts occur as the oedematous infarct enlarges squashing the surrounding normal brain against the skull and away from the core of the infarct causing herniation and midline shifts in severe cases. Swelling in the posterior fossa often leads to hydrocephalus (Fig. 3.28).

E~Stands for Evolution
The infarct must always be seen as an evolving lesion often with time-dependent consequences. The common outcome is for the swelling to resolve and the necrotic brain is phagocytosed and surrounding ischemic areas undergo apoptosis leaving behind a permanent low density on the CT as in Fig. 3.26. The other path of evolution is a hemorrhagic conversion which is illustrated Fig. 3.29. *'Acutely therefore the swelling can cause hydrocephalus, herniation or other catastrophic change that may be immediately fatal, hence the last thing you look for on the CT scan is for any of these complications of the CVA.'*

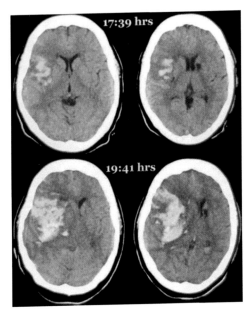

FIGURE 3.29. Non-contrast CT scan of a 60-year-old lady with sudden left hemiplegia who had thrombolysis. Immediate CT scan prior to thrombolysis was unremarkable (not shown) Six hours following thrombolysis, the CT scan at 17:39 h was obtained for increased drowsiness. Two hours later, large increase in the size of the clot is evident, *'this hemorrhagic conversion can occur with or without thrombolysis.'*

Although this chapter has summarized this very complex area of neuroimaging, it is hoped that some understanding of the basic principles and relevant attitudes can be cultivated from the approach outlined here. *'The golden rule which is worth repeating here is that – the CT scan is only an adjunct to the clinical assessment and not the main source of management decisions!'*

Chapter 4
Hydrocephalus

INTRODUCTION

'*The basic approach to all hydrocephalus is the same: you have to make a judgement whether the size of the ventricles is "normal" or not, for the individual patient*.' However, two broad groups of patients can be identified when looking for hydrocephalus in a brain CT scan in everyday clinical practice. The first group of patients are those whose hydrocephalus had **already** been **diagnosed** (hence they may have previous scans to compare with) and the second group are those patients that have had **no previous imaging before**. We will consider the second group first. Ventricular enlargement when gross is very easy to recognize on the CT scan (Fig. 4.1A), **but the key question is whether it is under high pressure or not because hydrocephalus technically is ventriculomegaly associated with raised intracranial pressure.**

It would have been nice if all cases of hydrocephalus were this obvious; however, there are a few basic principles that can be applied to make the majority of cases as obvious as this one. The first important clue is to grasp the layout of the ventricles and the pathway of CSF flow and hence the **sites prone to obstruction**.

The lateral ventricle consists of frontal horn, the body, occipital horn and the temporal horns (Fig. 4.2A and C). The **bodies** of the two lateral ventricles are only separated by a thin membrane, the *septum pellucidum*, so they practically touch in the midline. The third ventricle, cerebral aqueduct of Sylvius and the fourth ventricle are in the midline leaving the final shape of the ventricles like the drawing in Fig. 4.3.

U. Igbaseimokumo, *Brain CT Scans in Clinical Practice*,
DOI 10.1007/b98343_4, © Springer-Verlag London Limited 2009

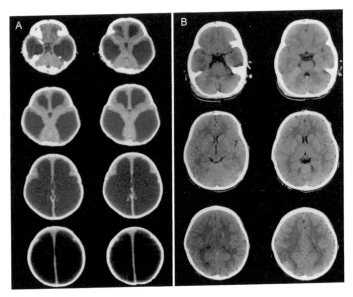

FIGURE 4.1. Non-contrast CT scan of an infant with massive hydro-cephalus with little cortical mantle (A). Note that in the normal CT scan (B), the third ventricle is slit like and the temporal horns are not easily seen at all and you *can* see the Sylvian fissure easily in spite of the large cortical mantle compared to A where the Sylvian fissure and the sulci are effaced (squashed up).

THE TEMPORAL HORNS AND THIRD VENTRICLE IN EARLY HYDROCEPHALUS

Not all cases of hydrocephalus are like Fig. 4.1(A) that are self evident as soon as you look at the CT scan. Determining the presence of hydrocephalus in less obvious cases therefore requires a systematic approach, and the first important clue to early hydrocephalus is enlargement of the temporal horns. Because the temporal horns are only barely visible (if at all) in the normal scan, their ready visualization is a cue to search for other evidence of ventricular enlargement. Figure 4.4 shows temporal horn enlargement as evidence of early hydrocephalus. Look for temporal horns in the slices near the base of the skull in the temporal lobe!

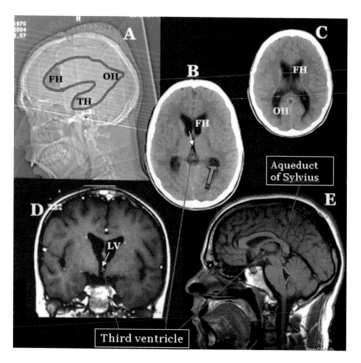

FIGURE 4.2. (A) Planning tomogram of the skull with the outline of the *lateral ventricle* superimposed in red. (B) and (C) Axial non-contrast brain CT scan showing lateral ventricles, frontal horns (FH), occipital horn (OH), the foramen of Munro (white arrow), and the thick green arrow is pointing down into the left temporal horn. The coronal MRI (D) emphasizes how the CSF flows from the lateral ventricles through the foramen of Munro (white arrow) on either side into the third ventricle (compare with Fig. 4.2B). Note that the foramen of Munro is just like a hallway that opens from the lateral ventricle into the third. From the third ventricle, CSF flows to the fourth ventricle (blue outline in Fig. 4.2E) through the narrow aqueduct of Sylvius. (FH = frontal horn; TH = temporal horn; OH = occipital horn; LV = lateral ventricle).

The next important clue, which is also evident in Fig. 4.4, is that the third ventricle which normally presents a narrow slit like appearance (Fig. 4.5A) changes to an oval shape, and in late cases to a frankly rounded third ventricle indicating severe hydrocephalus (Fig. 4.5D). Thus enlargement of the third ventricle is the second reliable sign of active hydrocephalus in the CT scan.

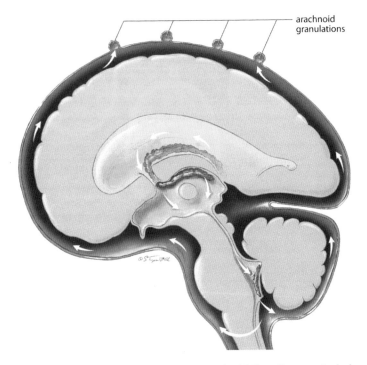

arachnoid
granulations

FIGURE 4.3. Model of ventricular system and CSF flow. Note particularly that CSF is produced as an ultrafiltrate of plasma in the choroids plexus located in the lateral, third and fourth ventricles. CSF leaves the ventricular system through the foramen of Magendie (midline inferiorly) and the foramina of Luschka in either lateral angle of the fourth ventricle. From here the CSF enters the subarachnoid space at the base of the skull distributing to the lumbar sac and also flows from the base towards the vertex of the brain where it is absorbed back into the blood at the arachnoid granulations. When hydrocephalus is the result of obstruction of the intraventricular CSF pathways then it is called ***obstructive hydrocephalus.*** However, if the CSF actually leaves the foramina of Luschka and Magendie and absorption is defective at the arachnoid villi in the subarachnoid space, then the hydrocephalus is called ***communicating:*** for instance, there is communication with the subarachnoid space. The importance of this distinction is that obstructive hydrocephalus develops relatively acutely due to the limited compliance from the ventricles. However, once the CSF communicates with the subarachnoid space, the compliance is greater and the onset of hydrocephalus is more gradual. '*In general the severity and rapidity of onset of symptoms is related to whether there is complete rapid obstruction or a slow gradual partial obstruction. But enlarged ventricles always call for detailed scrutiny by a more senior staff especially if a shunt is in place.*'

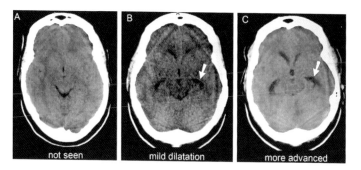

FIGURE 4.4. This figure illustrates increasing degrees of temporal horn dilatation in the same patient, a 40-year-old female school teacher with normal ventricles when the temporal horns were virtually invisible (A) and when she had early dilatation of the temporal horns due to subarachnoid hemorrhage (B). The final image (C) shows the same lady's CT scan when she developed more severe hydrocephalus due to cerebellar infarction. The significance of mild degrees of ventricular dilatation is often evident when considered with the clinical history or *previous films as in this case.*

EFFACEMENT OF THE SULCI

In addition to the above two important features, careful examination of the CT scans in Figs. 4.6 and 4.7 will show that the sulci are readily visible in Fig. 4.6 in spite of the enlarged ventricles. But in Fig. 4.7 only the large ventricles are the fluid spaces that are clearly visible and the sulci are completely indiscernible. As the ventricles enlarge with CSF under pressure, the brain is squeezed with the result that the gyri come together as shown in Fig. 1.10 (above) emptying the subarachnoid spaces (sulci) of CSF (and the sulci are said to be effaced – for instance not visible on the CT scan). This is a good indication of raised pressure within the ventricular cavity suggesting that the large ventricles are not due to passive dilatation due to loss of brain tissue (cerebral atrophy) but the result of forced enlargement like as if someone had blown water into a balloon (the brain).

DISPROPORTIONATELY SMALL FOURTH VENTRICLE

Also evident in Fig. 4.7 is the fact that the fourth ventricle appears disproportionately smaller in size compared to the size of the

Different degrees of hydrocephalus from normal to gross
Note third ventricle!

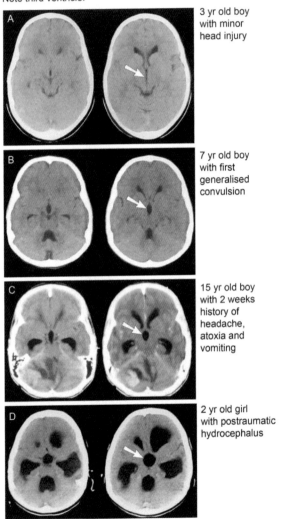

3 yr old boy
with minor
head injury

7 yr old boy
with first
generalised
convulsion

15 yr old boy
with 2 weeks
history of
headache,
atoxia and
vomiting

2 yr old girl
with postraumatic
hydrocephalus

FIGURE 4.5. Non-contrast brain CT scans showing different degrees of hydrocephalus: (A) Normal, (B) Mild hydrocephalus, (C) Moderately severe hydrocephalus, (D) Gross hydrocephalus (see text).

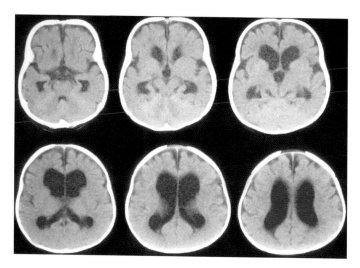

FIGURE 4.6. Non-contrast brain CT scan of an infant showing enlarged ventricles and prominent sulci suggesting some degree of cerebral atrophy. Note in particular that the subarachnoid spaces in the Sylvian fissures and over the frontal lobes are readily seen (compare with Fig. 4.7).

lateral and third ventricles. It suggests that the fourth ventricle is not dilated, which means the obstruction to CSF flow is before (proximal) to the fourth ventricle. It is an insight that comes readily with seeing many CT scans so I strongly suggest you pay attention to the size and shape of the fourth as you look at CT scans. We will come back to this in the next session on the causes of hydrocephalus. Figure 4.7 is a case of aqueduct stenosis presenting in later life.

THE FRONTAL AND OCCIPITAL HORNS

By far the larger and more prominent part of the ventricular system is the body of the lateral ventricle with the associated frontal and occipital horns. It is variable in size and highly susceptible to the effects of cerebral atrophy. For instance, cerebral atrophy leads to ex-vacuo dilatation of the ventricles in both children and adults. Comparison of Figs. 4.6 and 4.7 on the one hand with

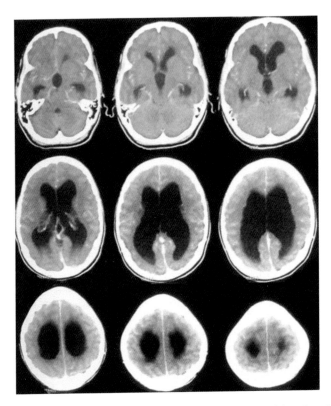

FIGURE 4.7. Non-contrast brain CT scan of a 22-year-old male with 3 weeks history of headaches and blurring of vision. Note the gross dilatation of the lateral ventricles (*the frontal horn, the body, occipital horn and temporal horns*) and the third ventricle. The sulci are effaced (see text).

Figs. 4.8 and 4.9 illustrates the changes in the body of the lateral ventricle in hydrocephalus. Note that Fig. 4.8 represents normal (but significant) variations in the size of the lateral ventricles as in the two children illustrated here.

In hydrocephalus, the frontal and occipital horns become rounded in shape and larger than the normal variations illustrated in Figs. 4.8 and 4.9. A case of gross severe hydrocephalus is illustrated in Fig. 4.10, which shows the obvious enlargement and the rounded nature of the OH and FH in hydrocephalus in addition to illustrating periventricular lucencies.

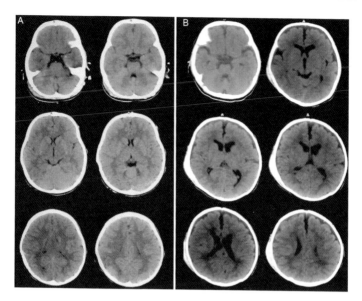

FIGURE 4.8. Non-contrast CT scan showing normal variations in the size of the lateral ventricles of two children (A) and (B). Note that in spite of the larger lateral ventricles in Fig. 4.8(B), the occipital horns remain narrow and the third ventricle shows no signs of ballooning out and the temporal horns remain small making this a normal variant.

PERIVENTRICULAR LUCENCIES

In Fig. 4.10, the white matter next to the frontal horns appears darker than it is elsewhere, giving the visual image of a teddy-bear with an ill-fitting small cap. That dark cap over the frontal horn is a sign of very late and severe hydrocephalus. *'There are few exceptions but suffice it to say that it is safe to always treat this as evidence of severe hydrocephalus until proven otherwise.'* So the appropriate action will be to make sure a neurosurgeon evaluate the patient and the scan.

With the above steps, you will most likely be able to make a judgement on whether the ventricles are enlarged or not in the majority of cases and if the pressure in the ventricles is raised.

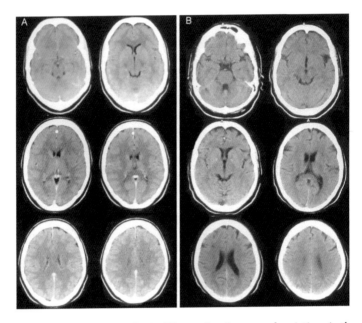

FIGURE 4.9. Non-contrast brain CT scan showing normal variations in the size of the lateral ventricles of two adults (A) and (B). Similar to Fig. 4.8B, the adult CT with larger ventricles (Fig. 4.9B) also shows narrow occipital and frontal horns along with readily visible sulci making this a normal variant. Compare with Fig. 4.7 in which the FH and OH are rounded in appearance and the sulci are effaced.

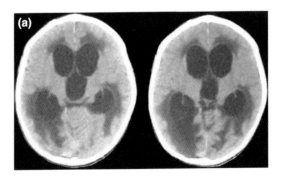

FIGURE 4.10A. Non-contrast brain CT scan showing severe hydrocephalus characterized by the ballooned (Mickey mouse shaped) ventricles with periventricular lucencies (white arrows). Note also the effacement of the sulci due to the grossly dilated ventricles.

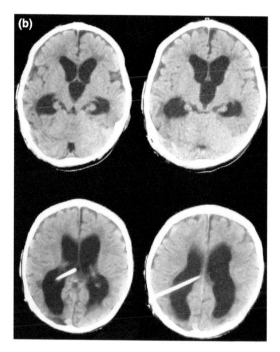

FIGURE 4.10B. The same patient following a successful ventriculoperitoneal shunt. The periventricular lucencies have disappeared and the sulci are clearly visible under the skull. The ***ventricles*** are smaller than in Fig. 4.10A and not under pressure anymore.

PREVIOUSLY DIAGNOSED HYDROCEPHALUS

The next group of patients are those with a ventriculoperitoneal shunt (or previously treated hydrocephalus, e.g. third ventriculostomy or excision of posterior fossa tumor). The systematic approach to looking at the CT scan is exactly the same except that you have the advantage and ***responsibility*** to obtain the previous imaging and compare with the present CT scan to see if the ventricles are bigger (Fig. 4.11A and B). It helps to focus in the same areas like the temporal horns and the third ventricle and then the lateral ventricles, comparing the new CT scan with the very last scan when the patient was well. Although comparison with previous imaging makes any changes in ventricular size obvious, it is important to realize that if such imaging is not available then

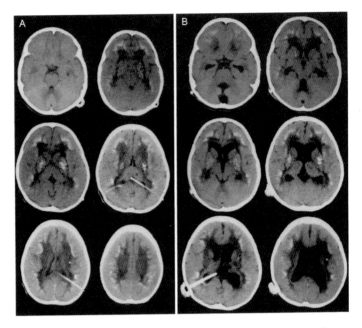

FIGURE 4.11. Non-contrast brain CT scan showing two scans from a patient with a ventriculoperitoneal shunt. It is important to note that there is pan ventricular dilatation in (B) with obvious dilatation of the temporal horns and third ventricle. In less obvious cases, detailed comparison of the scans is essential.

the same principles outlined above should be used to evaluate the current brain CT scan.

CAUSES OF HYDROCEPHALUS

Although it is true that hydrocephalus is always secondary to some underlying pathology or anomaly, from a practical point of view it is important to determine if there is only a CSF flow obstruction as in aqueduct stenosis or there is another serious underlying pathology like a tumour or a clot that may require treatment in its own right. Thus the final question you ask yourself after you see evidence of hydrocephalus on the CT scan is this: *'what is the cause of the hydrocephalus?'* Figure 4.7 is an example of aqueduct stenosis so that relieving the CSF obstruction results in cure. However, the enhancing (white) cerebellar tumour in Fig. 4.5C above is the primary diagnosis and the hydrocephalus is the secondary effect, a concept worth keeping in mind as you study the following cases in which the hydrocephalus is only part of the diagnosis and the underlying cause should be emphasized.

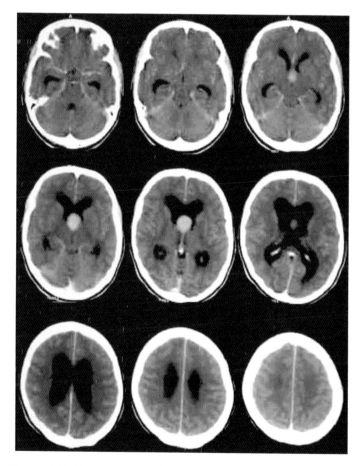

FIGURE 4.12. Post-contrast axial CT scan showing an anterior third ventricle colloid cyst blocking both foramina of Munro and causing severe hydrocephalus. Note that the third and fourth ventricles are small or normal because the obstruction is proximal to this level.

It is beyond the scope of this book to detail all the possible causes of hydrocephalus from the choroids plexus to the dural venous sinuses, therefore only striking illustrations will be given but the concept ought to be clear that hydrocephalus can occur from either CSF over production (choroids plexus papilloma) or reduced absorption. The reduced absorption can either be from obstruction or other mechanisms. By and large the majority of cases are from obstruction, which is secondary to either a congenital lesion, tumour, hemorrhage or infection. Fortunately these are easy to differentiate from the history and physical examination and a review of the brain CT scan.

Foramen of Munro – Colloid Cyst
A colloid cyst is a classic example at this location and is illustrated in Fig. 4.12. The third ventricle remains small or normal as the obstruction is upstream. However when the obstruction is either in the aqueduct of sylvius (Fig. 4.13) or in the fourth ventricle (Fig. 4.14) the third ventricle enlarges significantly.

Cerebral Aqueduct of Sylvius

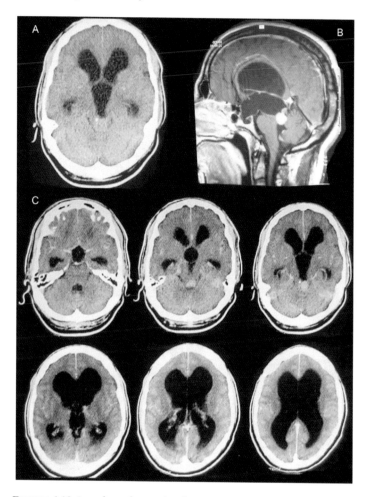

FIGURE 4.13 Aqueduct obstruction from pineocytoma. A= non-contrast axial CT; B= sagittal post-contrast MRI showing the enhancing nodule of tumour causing the obstruction; C= post-contrast CT scan showing the enhancing nodule as seen on CT. Note that the third ventricle is larger than the fourth a reversal of the normal situation, which is the hallmark of aqueduct stenosis (compare Fig. 4.7) no matter the cause.

Fourth Ventricle Obstruction

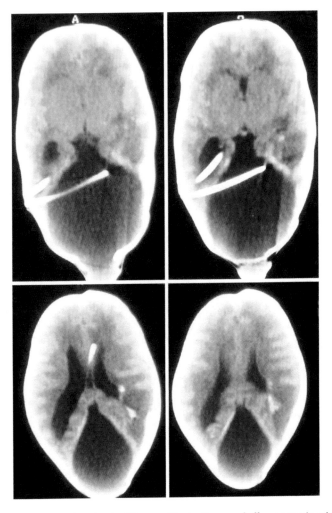

FIGURE 4.14. Infant brain CT scan illustrating cerebellar agenesis with large Dandy Walker cyst causing hydrocephalus. *'Fourth ventricle or its exit foramina can be obstructed by a Dandy Walker cyst as in this case or tumour or swollen cerebellum from CVA or adhesions from infection or haematoma resulting in hydrocephalus.'*

Chapter 5
Tumours and Infections (☞ SOL)

INTRODUCTION

Brain tumours and abscesses (which most physicians refer to collectively as space-occupying lesions – SOL) exert a significant mass effect on the brain. In addition, most radiologists would recall trying to differentiate a tumour from an abscess and vice versa. The distinction is *critical* for obvious reasons – a brain tumour like a glioblastoma is effectively a terminal illness whereas most bacterial abscesses are curable with antibiotics and drainage. It is to emphasize this distinction and the urgency to come to a conclusion in both cases that we are discussing these two subjects in the same chapter. By and large both lesions will present with one or more of the following clinical problems: features of raised ICP, convulsions, headache, focal neurological deficit (like hemiparesis or speech disturbance) plus or minus altered level of consciousness. Fever is variable even in brain abscesses. Slow-growing tumours may give rise to a longer duration of symptoms.

In the preceding chapters, we have simply discussed obvious lesions with little need for differential diagnosis. Tumours such as meningiomas (Fig. 5.8) are again obvious and call for little differential diagnosis. However, the majority of metastatic tumours and intrinsic high-grade gliomas, which together make up the majority of tumours seen in emergency medicine may need to be distinguished from an abscess (Fig. 5.1A and B). We will try and simplify this process so that you can deal with the 80% or more of the straightforward cases without feeling turned into a neuro-radiologist! Let us look at the basics of describing any tumour or abscess, which I have reduced to the acronym MEAL. (Well, we will try not to *make a meal of it!*)

U. Igbaseimokumo, *Brain CT Scans in Clinical Practice*, DOI 10.1007/b98343_5, © Springer-Verlag London Limited 2009

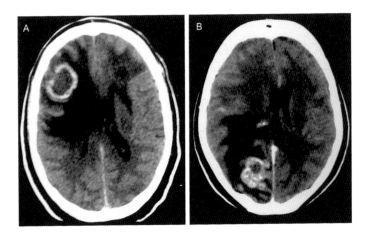

Figure 5.1. (A) and (B) are post-contrast CT scans showing two obvious lesions. One is a tuberculosis granuloma and the other a metastatic lung carcinoma. This picture is intended to reinforce the not infrequent similarity between tumours and infective lesions. What is your guess as to which is tumour and which is TB? See below for the answer.

M IS FOR MASS EFFECT

The concept of mass effect was introduced in Chapter 1. Comparing the appearance of the sulci and gyri between the two sides (right and left) of the brain makes any differences apparent. (If you have any doubt about the appearance of gyri and sulci on the CT scan, then this is a good time to revise chapter one especially Figs. 1.10, 1.11, 1.12 and 1.15). The side with a tumour or abscess is more likely to have the sulci squeezed (effaced) and often the lateral ventricle on that side is also compressed (Fig. 5.2A and C), and in more severe cases there is midline shift towards the normal side. This is often the first clue that there may be a lesion (Fig. 5.2A) prompting the intravenous injection of contrast (see below) to see if the lesion takes up contrast and become brighter. Review the examples in Fig. 5.2 and see if you can describe the abnormality in the CT scan in each case (A, B and C).

Although most brain tumours will declare their presence by a significant mass effect from their share *size* (Figs. 5.2A and C) or by the *severe oedema* around them (Fig. 5.3), other lesions show very little mass effect and are only picked up (identified) on close systematic scrutiny of all the images (Fig. 5.4 tumour without mass effect).

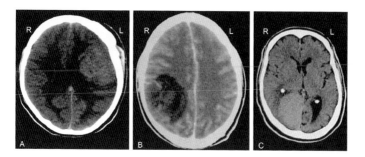

Figure 5.2. Non-contrast brain CT scan showing alterations of the normal sulcal pattern as evidence of mass effect from an isodense meningioma (A), a low-density glioma (B) and a hyperdense meningioma (C).

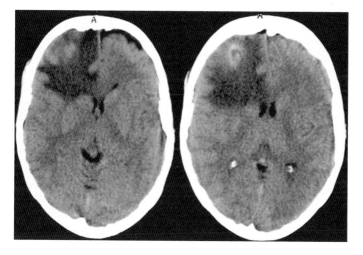

Figure 5.3. Non-contrast brain CT scan showing severe right frontal oedema with mass effect. The right frontal horn is effaced (not seen) whereas the left is clearly seen. The sulci and CSF subarachnoid spaces are more easily seen on the left than on the right and there is midline shift to the left seen more clearly in Fig. 5.3B.

E IS FOR ENHANCEMENT

"Enhancement simply means it is appearing clearer" and in this case higher density compared to the pre-contrast scan. Certain chemicals like iohexol (non-ionic) and diatrizoate (ionic) appear hyperdense on CT scan. When injected intravenously they

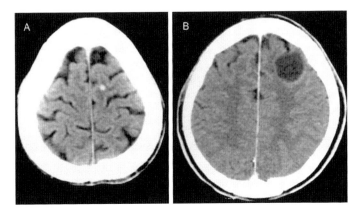

Figure 5.4. A and B are different patients with axial CT scans illustrating a small hyperdense lesion with no mass effect (A) and a larger left frontal low-grade glioma with little mass effect. Note that the sulci are clearly visible and almost undisturbed by the left frontal lesion (see white arrow).

concentrate in vascular areas of the brain including tumours and abscess walls thereby making them appear hyperdense and hence easier to see (for instance, enhancing their appearance Fig. 5.5, Fig. 5.8). The neovascular capillaries of tumours and the abscess wall are often porous allowing some of the contrast to leak into the interstitial area thereby accumulating in the tumour or abscess wall *for sufficiently long enough time to be imaged.* The time between the injection of contrast and CT imaging is important because with time the contrast gets washed out from the tumour by the blood so undue delay may lead to a *false appearance of lack of enhancement*.

Meningiomas and lymphomas tend to enhance uniformly and intensely whereas malignant gliomas and abscesses may show an intermediate degree of enhancement in which there is an outer enhancing ring surrounding a core of non-enhancing low density (necrotic centre), which fails to take up the contrast (Figs. 5.6 and 5.7). Abscesses (Fig. 5.6) typically show a *uniform, thin* enhancing wall surrounding the pus whereas the ring of enhancement in gliomas is thicker with more solid tumour in the wall (Fig. 5.7).

'In general abscesses have a thinner and smoother enhancing ring with no chunk of enhancing tumour along the wall. Whereas the enhancing ring in malignant gliomas and metastatic tumours tends to be thicker and irregular and there may be an asymmetric

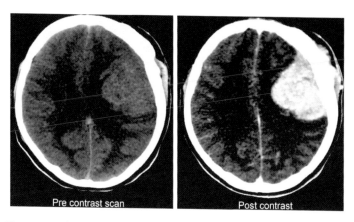

Figure 5.5. shows the pre- and post-contrast CT scans of a 22-year-old male that presented with his first grand mal fit. He admitted to having a large mass on the left side of his head for over one year. This history clearly suggests a slow-growing tumour like a meningioma. Identification of a mass lesion is so much easier if there is significant enhancement. The pre-contrast scan is same as in Fig. 5.2A. The effect of the contrast enhancement is obvious. Although the meningioma is iodense and can only be inferred from the mass effect (effacement of the sulci, compression of the left lateral ventricle and midline shift), the contrast enhancement makes it obvious.

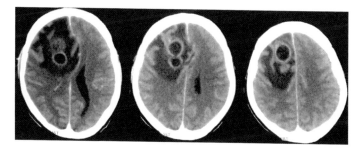

Figure 5.6. Contrast-enhanced brain CT scan showing a brain abscess in a 38-year-old man on immunesuppression therapy for SLE. Note the smooth outline of the rings of enhancement.

large chunk of enhancing tumour as part of the wall (Fig. 5.7).' By these descriptions, Fig. 5.1A should be an abscess and 88B a tumour but the **reverse** is true. Figure 5.1B was actually biopsied and confirmed to be a tuberculosis granuloma, which

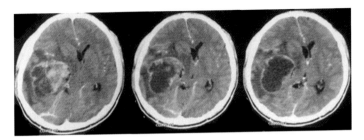

Figure 5.7. Contrast-enhanced brain CT scan showing right temporal gliobastoma in a 21-year-old male with first grand mal seizure. Note the solid mass of enhancing tissue, the cystic non-enhancing core and the severe mass effect with effacement of the right lateral ventricle and midline shift. This requires urgent neurosurgical referral due to significant midline shift and brain compression.

disappeared completely with antituberculous treatment and 88A was confirmed a metastatic tumour from the lung. Unfortunately such exceptions to the general description given here are common, because the similarity between brain abscesses and malignant tumours is not only in appearance but the result of their

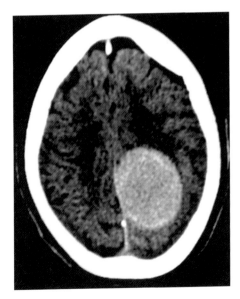

Figure 5.8.
Contrast-enhanced
brain CT scan
illustrating a uniformly
enhancing left
parafalcine
meningioma. Note that
it is solid and very
unlike an abscess. It is
benign and carries a
good prognosis.

common biological aggressiveness in destroying everything in their path as they advance into the surrounding brain like an invading army. The result is often the same – *death and destruction* – no matter the 'regiment[1]' carrying it out! Thus malignant gliomas and abscesses both leave necrotic tissue on their imperial path, hence the similar appearance. '*So it has to be emphasized that for the frontline doctor, an accurate description of the lesion is far better than histological exactitude from the CT scan.*'

You should note carefully that tumours like meningioma do not look like abscesses and are therefore not easily confused.

Malignant gliomas and metastatic tumours *share* the property of ring enhancement with abscesses and are therefore the subject of much clinical controversy. '*From a frontline physician's point of view describing accurately what the lesion looks like on the emergency contrast-enhanced CT scan to a neurosurgeon is more than adequate and it will be the responsibility of the neurosurgeon and neuroradiologist to consider the differential diagnosis.*' For the anxious patient and relative, the frontline doctor simply have to be honest and say that the exact nature of the mass lesion can only be confirmed after a biopsy and guessing is unwise – which is true as exceptions are common (Fig. 5.1). However, it is imperative for the physician to be able to say if there is significant mass effect or immediate risk to life based on the presence or absence of the specific features discussed in the section on *red flags.*

Enhancement is a common feature of infective lesions. Most brain abscesses (pyogenic and granulomatous) will show ring enhancement when a mature abscess exists. The difference between a subdural haematoma and empyema (Fig. 5.9) may well depend on the presence or absence of how vivid the enhancement is, if the clinical features are equivocal. And in meningitis, the meninges show widespread enhancement. Thus the presence or absence of enhancement should be evaluated carefully. Having raised your awareness to think of metastasis, glioma and abscess when you have a ring-enhancing tumour, it is important to point out that both metastasis and gliomas could appear as solid tumours prior to the formation of a necrotic centre. Again the emphasis should be to determine if there is any mass effect and if the lesion poses immediate risk to life (see red flags below) rather than the accuracy of the differential diagnosis.

---

[1]Cancer or bacteria

Figure 5.9.
Contrast brain
CT scan
showing the
enhancing rim
surrounding a
subdural
empyema.

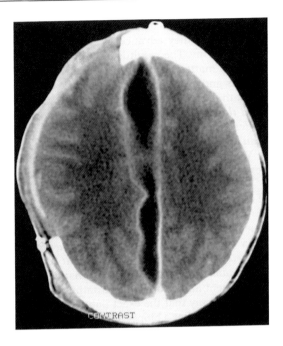

A IS FOR APPEARANCE

Appearance simply means what does it look like? What is the shape of the mass or tumour you have seen? Usually the pre- and post-contrast films should be examined, and as much as possible avoid trying to describe a scan from memory. Always have the films in front of you, when you are trying to describe it to someone on the phone or write down a comment in the patient's file. The first thing you notice about the appearance of any lesion is whether it is hyperdense, isodense or hypodense on the pre-contrast film. Note that hyperdense lesions imply blood or calcification. Hypodense lesions usually signify oedema or fluid. The post-contrast film is then scrutinized to determine the shape of the enhancing component. '*A uniform enhancement implies a solid mass like a meningioma (Fig. 5.8); a patchy irregular enhancement will suggest a partially solid and cystic tumour like a glioma (Fig. 5.10) and a ring enhancing, circular lesion (Fig. 5.11) will suggest an abscess with the important differential diagnosis of a metastasis or glioma.*'

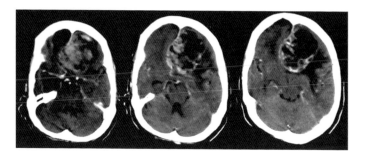

Figure 5.10. Contrast CT scan showing a left frontal irregularly enhancing tumour with solid and cystic components. This is a typical appearance for a high-grade glioma usually glioblastoma.

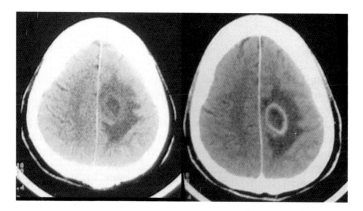

Figure 5.11. Pre- and post-contrast CT scan showing a left parietal ring-enhancing lesion with surrounding oedema (low-density area). Stereotactic aspiration showed a Nocardia brain abscess.

L IS FOR LOCATION

Sixty percent of primary tumours in adults are supratentorial and 40% occur in the posterior fossa. The reverse is true for children: for instance, 60% posterior fossa and 40% supratentorial. One of the critical factors about the location of a tumour is the propensity for complications. Colloid cysts in the third ventricle typically cause hydrocephalus (Fig. 4.12) and may result in sudden death from unrecognized and acutely progressively raised ICP from CSF flow obstruction. A tumour in the temporal lobe frequently

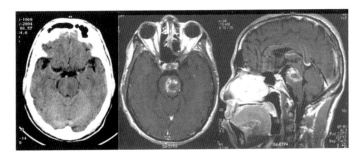

Figure 5.12. The CT scan on the left hardly gives any clue of the fatal brain stem glioma easily displayed by the MRI. *'If the patient has obvious clinical signs and symptoms then you must scrutinize the image for the hidden clue, which here is the enlarged pons and central low density. Remember to have a contrast enhanced film!'*.

presents with epilepsy and easily compresses the brain stem. Posterior fossa tumours often cause hydrocephalus (Fig. 4.5C). So the location is important and is one vital piece of information the neurosurgeon may want to know at the end of the phone. It is perhaps superfluous at this stage to emphasize that it is imperative to note whether the lesion is in the left or right hemisphere and which part of the brain – frontal, parietal, temporal or cerebellum or brain stem. Brain stem lesions are often difficult to see unless the clinical history leads you to search carefully (Fig. 5.12).

Brain tumours broadly occur in *two layers:* those tumours arising from and located in intimate contact with the coverings of the brain including the skull base (such as meningiomas) versus those that are located within the substance of the brain itself (such as gliomas and metastasis). Although there are many exceptions such that large gliomas may come to the surface touching the skull (Fig. 5.13); meningiomas however arise from the meninges and therefore tend to make broad contact with the dura (along the vault, the sphenoid wings and the falx cerebri) often displaying an enhancing tail that is typical of these tumours (Fig. 5.14). However, gliomas and metastasis generally have the epicentre of the tumour located in the white matter (Fig. 5.15) even if it extends to the surface. This basic fact from the CT scan applied correctly with other factors such as the appearance and enhancing characteristics will allow identification of the common tumour types even by a frontline doctor.

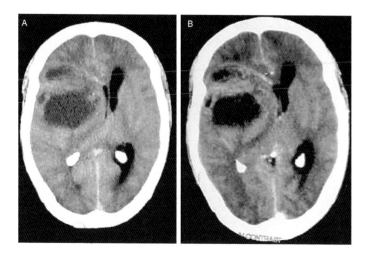

Figure 5.13. Contrast CT scan showing a moderately enhancing right fronto-parietal glioma coming to the surface. Note it is multicystic with a significant mass effect. The right frontal horn is completely squashed and there is midline shift to the left.

Thus if you describe a uniformly enhancing tumour with a broad based attachment to the dura, it is a meningioma until proven otherwise. If you describe a ring-enhancing lesion located deep in the white matter, you most likely have a glioblastoma or an abscess or a metastasis.

SPECIAL LOCATIONS

Tumours of the pituitary fossa and cerebellopontine angle often come with a suggestive history of visual failure and deafness respectively, which requires these areas to be scrutinized carefully. It is self evident how easy it is for a beginner to miss the pituitary tumour illustrated in Fig. 5.16. Furthermore small tumours in the posterior fossa may be missed either due to artefacts from the surrounding bones or lack of systematic evaluation of the posterior fossa in the CT scan (Fig. 5.12).

Although certain tumours occur in certain locations, and childhood tumours tend to differ from adult tumours, it is more important to describe accurately the lesion seen on the pre- and post-contrast CT scans rather than a pedantic assertion of tumour

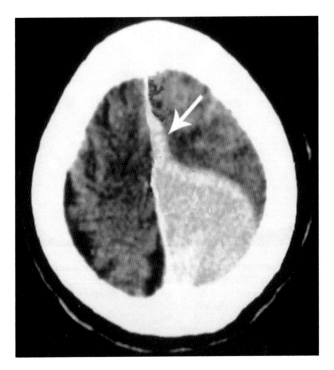

Figure 5.14. Contrast-enhanced CT scan showing a typical meningioma arising from the falx cerebri and manifesting an enhancing dural tail (the white arrow).

type, because CT radiological assessment of histological types or grade is at best imprecise. Therefore, the above summary is intended to give you the tools with which to describe a tumour or any mass lesion accurately.

Red Flags

'The most important indication for urgent action is the degree of mass effect, which is often related to the size of the tumour or abscess. Significant midline shift over 5 mm, contralateral hydrocephalus and tumours compressing the brain stem constitute high-risk features. The most important red flag however is the clinical state of the patient – presence or absence of any alteration in level of consciousness and papillary changes constitute strong indicators for intervention as the brain scan.'

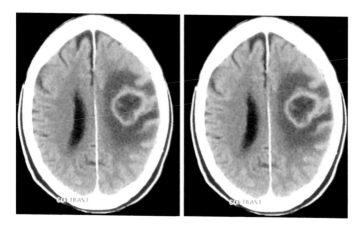

Figure 5.15. Post-contrast scans showing a typical left frontal glioblastoma multiformi, which is centred in the white mater with surrounding oedema coming to the surface.

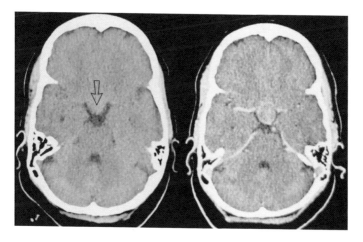

Figure 5.16. Pre- and post-contrast scans showing a pituitary adenoma.

Chapter 6
Advanced Uses of Brain CT Scan

3D RENDITIONS: CRANIOSYNOSTOSIS

In paediatrics, 3D rendition of the skull gives incredibly beautiful and confirmatory pictures of the skull bones in cases of craniosynostosis. In Fig. 6.1, a metopic synostosis with the front of the head narrowed into a triangular peak (trigonocephaly) is illustrated. Special uses like these are only limited by the dose of radiation necessary to obtain this quality of pictures.

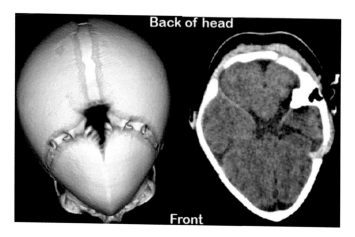

FIGURE 6.1. 3D scan of the skull showing fused metopic suture.

U. Igbaseimokumo, *Brain CT Scans in Clinical Practice*,
DOI 10.1007/b98343_6, © Springer-Verlag London Limited 2009

3D RENDITIONS: CT ANGIOGRAPHY

Although digital substraction angiography as we saw in Fig. 3.15 remains the gold standard, increasingly sophisticated CT imaging protocols allow the visualization of the cerebral vessels (CT angiography) in 3 dimensions (Fig. 6.2) providing useful information and in some centres obviating the need for standard angiography.

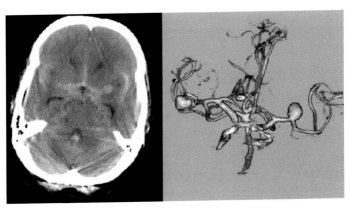

FIGURE 6.2. Plain CT scan showing subarachnoid hemorrhage and a 3D CT angiogram showing multiple aneurysms (left and right middle cerebral artery aneurysms – round blebs on the arterial tree like pumpkins and an ACOM aneurysm).

SUBTLETIES!

Confirming your assessment of the CT scan with the radiologists' report represents both opportunity to learn and good practice. There will always be scans that challenge even the expert and you never know when one such scan will come calling. Use the principles you have learnt here but do not hesitate to ask for help.

The scans below (Fig. 6.3) belong to a child who suffered non-accidental trauma from his carer on the 29th of November. The CT scan one month later show hyperdense white matter, but the grey matter is isodense with overlying subdural collection. An experienced radiologist had trouble telling the end of the cortex (brain) and the subdural. The follow-up scan from January with the catheter makes it clear that the darkness beyond the white

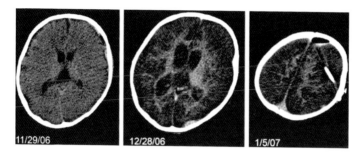

FIGURE 6.3. Serial CT scans showing evolution of encephalomalacia.

matter consists of subdural effusion and brain cortex, almost completely indistinguishable. The catheter is on the surface of the brain not intraparenchymal. Such an appearance will confuse experts and beginners alike. In addition there is emerging technology that will daunt even the greatest enthusiast. This introduction is therefore to get you started, a solid foundation to build on.

Index